Cytotoxicity - Definition, Identification, and Cytotoxic Compounds

*Edited by Erman Salih Istifli
and Hasan Basri Ila*

Published in London, United Kingdom

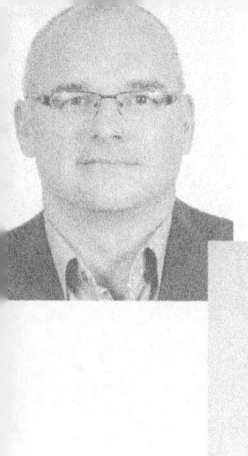
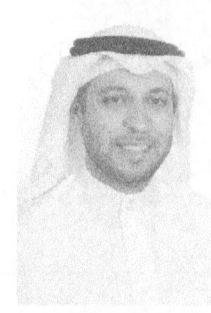
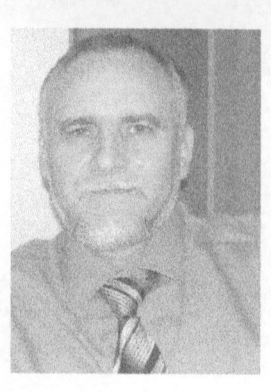
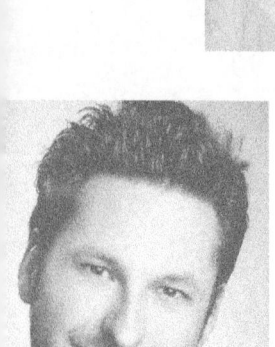
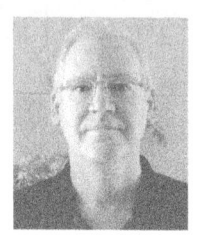
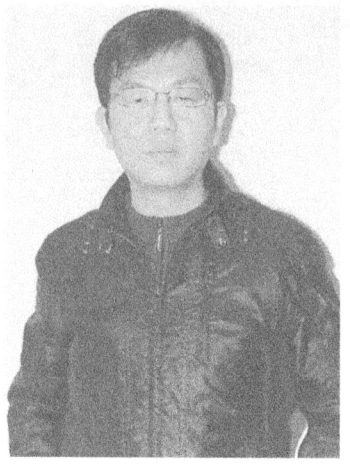
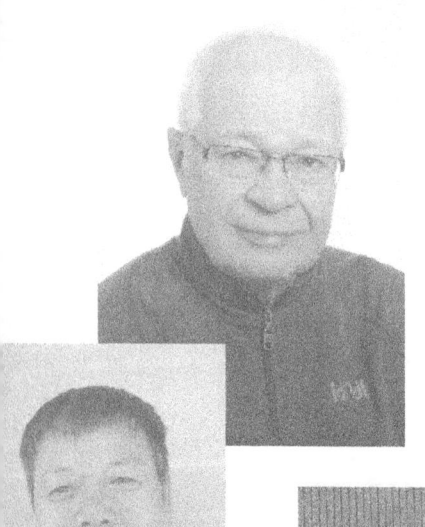
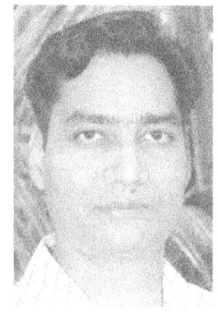
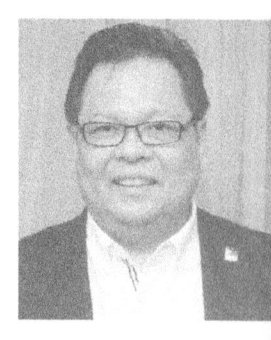
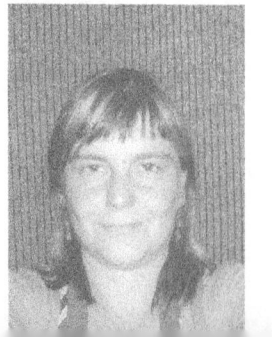
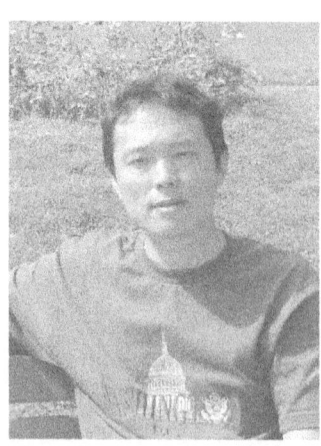

IntechOpen

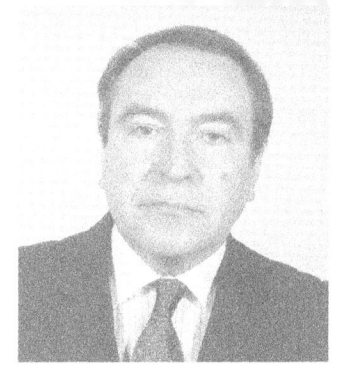
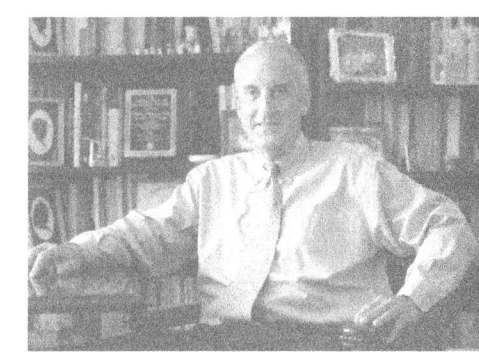
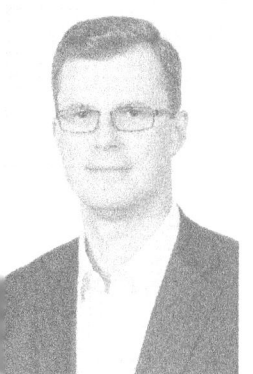
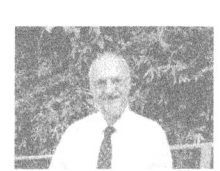
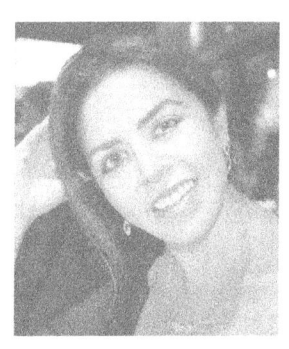

Supporting open minds since 2005

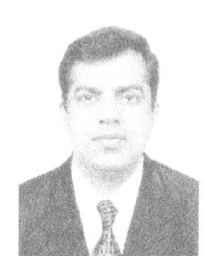
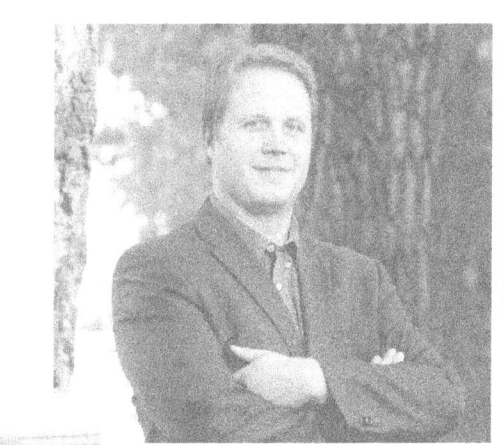
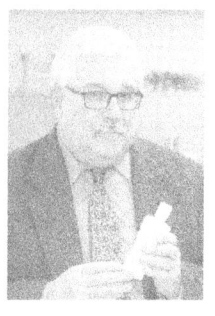
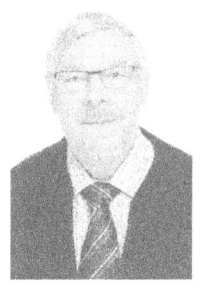
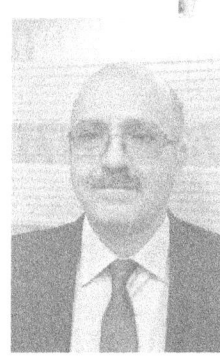
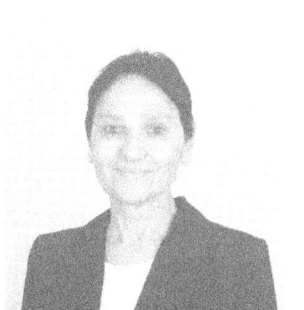
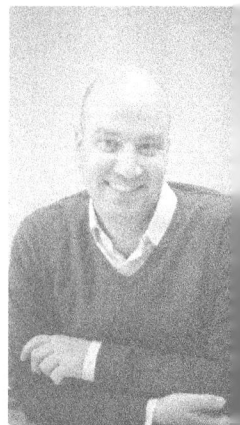

Cytotoxicity - Definition, Identification, and Cytotoxic Compounds
http://dx.doi.org/10.5772/intechopen.77899
Edited by Erman Salih Istifli and Hasan Basri Ila

Contributors
Khairan Khairan, Claus Jacob, Karl-Herbert Schaefer, Igor Okolov, Olga Aleksandrova, Juliya Khorolskaya, Natalia Mikhailova, Diana Darvish, Miralda Blinova, El-Shimaa Mohamed Naguib Abdel-Hafez, Mohamed Hassan, Sara Abdelhafez, Adel Abelhakeem, Salud Perez, Cuauhtémoc Pérez González, Julia Pérez Ramos, Carlos Alberto Méndez-Cuesta, Roberto José Serrano Vega, Miguel Martell Mendoza, Maria Del Consuelo Gómez, Crisalde Ramirez, Elvia Pérez, Cynthia Carolina Estanislao, Guillermo Pérez, Erman Salih Istifli

© The Editor(s) and the Author(s) 2019
The rights of the editor(s) and the author(s) have been asserted in accordance with the Copyright, Designs and Patents Act 1988. All rights to the book as a whole are reserved by INTECHOPEN LIMITED. The book as a whole (compilation) cannot be reproduced, distributed or used for commercial or non-commercial purposes without INTECHOPEN LIMITED's written permission. Enquiries concerning the use of the book should be directed to INTECHOPEN LIMITED rights and permissions department (permissions@intechopen.com).
Violations are liable to prosecution under the governing Copyright Law.

(cc) BY

Individual chapters of this publication are distributed under the terms of the Creative Commons Attribution 3.0 Unported License which permits commercial use, distribution and reproduction of the individual chapters, provided the original author(s) and source publication are appropriately acknowledged. If so indicated, certain images may not be included under the Creative Commons license. In such cases users will need to obtain permission from the license holder to reproduce the material. More details and guidelines concerning content reuse and adaptation can be found at http://www.intechopen.com/copyright-policy.html.

Notice
Statements and opinions expressed in the chapters are these of the individual contributors and not necessarily those of the editors or publisher. No responsibility is accepted for the accuracy of information contained in the published chapters. The publisher assumes no responsibility for any damage or injury to persons or property arising out of the use of any materials, instructions, methods or ideas contained in the book.

First published in London, United Kingdom, 2019 by IntechOpen
IntechOpen is the global imprint of INTECHOPEN LIMITED, registered in England and Wales, registration number: 11086078, The Shard, 25th floor, 32 London Bridge Street
London, SE19SG - United Kingdom
Printed in Croatia

British Library Cataloguing-in-Publication Data
A catalogue record for this book is available from the British Library

Additional hard and PDF copies can be obtained from orders@intechopen.com

Cytotoxicity - Definition, Identification, and Cytotoxic Compounds
Edited by Erman Salih Istifli and Hasan Basri Ila
p. cm.
Print ISBN 978-1-78984-754-3
Online ISBN 978-1-78984-755-0
eBook (PDF) ISBN 978-1-83962-286-1

We are IntechOpen,
the world's leading publisher of
Open Access books
Built by scientists, for scientists

4,300+
Open access books available

116,000+
International authors and editors

130M+
Downloads

151
Countries delivered to

Our authors are among the
Top 1%
most cited scientists

12.2%
Contributors from top 500 universities

WEB OF SCIENCE™

Selection of our books indexed in the Book Citation Index
in Web of Science™ Core Collection (BKCI)

Interested in publishing with us?
Contact book.department@intechopen.com

Numbers displayed above are based on latest data collected.
For more information visit www.intechopen.com

Meet the editors

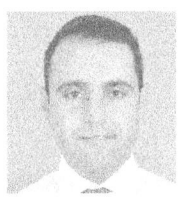

Dr. Erman Salih İstifli received his PhD from the Biology Department at Cukurova University, Insitute of Science and Letters. In his doctoral study, Dr. İstifli focused on the elucidation of the genotoxic and cytotoxic effects of a commonly used anticancer agent (antifolate) on human lymphocytes. Dr. İstifli, during his period of doctoral research, joined the molecular cytogenetics group at the Max Planck Institute for Molecular Genetics in Berlin, Germany, and he focused there on investigating the molecular cytogenetic causes of some human rare diseases. During these studies, he contributed experimentally to the identification of four candidate genes (GRIA2, GLRB, NPY1R, and NPY5R) responsible for intelligence and obesity. He was assigned as an expert and rapporteur on eight candidate projects in the Marie-Sklodowska Curie-Actions Innovative Training Networks in 2016. In 2017, he completed the online theoretical and practical course "Introduction to Biology - The Secret of Life," run by the Massachusetts Institute of Technology (MIT) on the edX platform. In April 2019, within the framework of Erasmus+ staff mobility program, he gave seminars on "DNA microarrays and their use in genotoxicity" at Tirana University in Tirana, Albania. In 2019, he was awarded a three-year Membership Certificate for UKRI (UK Research and Innovation) International Development Peer Review College. He is a published author of several articles in journals indexed by the SCI and SCI-E, and has manuscripts in other refereed scientific journals. He currently serves as a referee for several journals covered by the SCI and SCI-E. His studies mainly fall into the field of genetic toxicology.

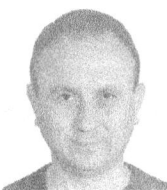

Prof. Dr. Hasan Basri İla received his PhD from the Biology Department at Çukurova University, Institute of Science and Letters. During his doctoral study, he investigated the effects of a commonly used antibiotic on chromosome aberration and micronucleus formation by in vivo tests. Dr. İla has several publications in internationally indexed (SCI, SCI-E) journals, and his articles have been cited 474 times. He has served as a researcher and project leader for 18 national projects. He gives lectures on biology, cytology, genetics, evolution, organelle genetics and cancer genetics. He has numerous poster and/or oral scientific presentations in several international conferences. He is co-editor of *Lymphocytes* published by IntechOpen in 2019. In the same year, he obtained a national patent on natural colorants isolated from the brideweed plant (*Bougainvillea glabra*).

Contents

Preface   XI

Section 1
Cytotoxicity Research   1

Chapter 1   3
In Vitro Cytotoxicity Screening as a Criterion for the Rational Selection of Tear Substitutes
by Olga I. Aleksandrova, Igor N. Okolov, Julia I. Khorolskaya, Natalia A. Mikhailova, Diana M. Darvish and Miralda I. Blinova

Chapter 2   15
Study of the Cytotoxic Activity of Haarlem Oil on Different Cell Lines and a Higher Organism, *Steinernema feltiae*
by Khairan Khairan, Torsten Burkholz, Mareike Kelkel, Vincent Jamier, Karl-Herbert Schäfer and Claus Jacob

Chapter 3   29
Cytotoxic Activity of Essential Oils of Some Species from Lamiaceae Family
by Cuauhtémoc Pérez-González, Julia Pérez-Ramos, Carlos Alberto Méndez-Cuesta, Roberto Serrano-Vega, Miguel Martell-Mendoza and Salud Pérez-Gutiérrez

Chapter 4   45
Cytotoxic Effect and Mechanisms from Some Plant-Derived Compounds in Breast Cancer
by Elvia Pérez-Soto, Cynthia Carolina Estanislao-Gómez, David Guillermo Pérez-Ishiwara, Crisalde Ramirez-Celis and María del Consuelo Gómez-García

Chapter 5   69
Apoptotic Inhibitors as Therapeutic Targets for Cell Survival
by El-Shimaa Mohamed Naguib Abdelhafez, Sara Mohamed Naguib Abdelhafez Ali, Mohamed Ramadan Eisa Hassan and Adel Mohammed Abdel-Hakem

Section 2
Methods in Cytotoxicity Assessment   85

Chapter 6   87
Cell Division, Cytotoxicity, and the Assays Used in the Detection of
Cytotoxicity
by Erman Salih Istifli, Mehmet Tahir Hüsunet and Hasan Basri Ila

Preface

Cell death by endogenous and/or exogenous effects is called cytotoxicity and the effect that leads to cell death is called the cytotoxic effect. The cytotoxic effect may be physical, chemical or biological.

The basic pathway in the reality of cytotoxicity is determined by the pattern by which the cell dies. Accordingly, the cell either attempts to die in a multi-step manner in the presence of a genetically controlled mechanism, which is called apoptosis (programmed cell death), or dies by a necrosis-like mechanism (without genetic control) that suddenly occurs for unpredictable reasons leading to inflammation.

Although not genetically controlled, some exogenous effects may also trigger apoptosis by reprogramming the genetic control of the cell-killing mechanism. There have been numerous examples of this phenomenon in practice, such as in conventional chemotherapy and radiotherapy.

The most important thing to consider at this point is, in fact, why the cell attempts to die in a controlled behaviour. This cellular death process in the organism is governed by various intrinsic purposes. One of these is the programmed destruction of a group of cells to facilitate morphogenesis during ontogenesis. Another is the pronounced cytotoxicity that takes place if the cell or subcellular compartments function insufficiently and/or are damaged.

From this perspective, *regeneration* is the reproduction of some cells that are somehow eliminated to maintain homeostasis in the organism. The first example of the use of the term regeneration in biology is seen in the example of Prometheus in Greek Mythology, who was tied to the rocks by Zeus for giving fire to the people of Mount Olympus. In this case, regeneration is observed as the constant renewal of Promethus' liver, which was fed to the eagles in order to increase the penalty. In this myth, the regeneration of the liver suggests any cell regeneration in the organism.

In any case, compensating for cytotoxicity in the multicellular organism by a certain level of cellular proliferation is the primary aim of homeostasis. In addition, the loss of cellular proliferation control (tumorigenesis) is at least as important as cytotoxicity, however, it is a contrasting trauma. With the disruption of the delicate balance between cytotoxicity and proliferation, confrontation with cancer can inevitably occur. As a result, a deep understanding of the molecular control of the mechanisms of cytotoxicity and cellular proliferation will be one of the most important perspectives in the struggle to stop cancer, the leading health problem of this century.

We hope this book will be an important and useful resource, especially for professional researchers and students studying cytotoxicity and its control.

Dr. Erman Salih Istifli and Dr. Hasan Basri Ila
Çukurova University,
Faculty of Science and Letters,
Department of Biology,
Adana, Turkey

Section 1
Cytotoxicity Research

Chapter 1

In Vitro Cytotoxicity Screening as a Criterion for the Rational Selection of Tear Substitutes

Olga I. Aleksandrova, Igor N. Okolov, Julia I. Khorolskaya, Natalia A. Mikhailova, Diana M. Darvish and Miralda I. Blinova

Abstract

A large number of artificial tears are currently available in the pharmaceutical market. Selecting the right drug for the patient remains a challenge for both the doctor and the patient. Comparing the cytotoxicity of artificial tears is one of the criteria for the rational selection of a drug that promotes maximum clinical efficacy and a higher safety profile. It is known that cells grown in vitro retain many metabolic features of the parent host tissues and at the same time lack tissue and organ interrelations and regulatory effects of the nervous and endocrine systems and have very limited compensatory capabilities. These features of cell cultures provide an opportunity to investigate the interaction of chemical agents directly with the cell itself, to identify changes in cellular and subcellular structures that can be masked in whole-organism settings. This study presents the results of assessing the cytotoxicity of tear substitutes, which demonstrate that these drugs can have a cytostatic effect in vitro and differ in their cytotoxic potential. In recent years, the problem of drug therapy of patients with dry eye syndrome has been attracting increasing attention of ophthalmologists, so screening the cytotoxicity of a wide range of tear substitutes using cell culture-based test systems can promote the rational selection of these drugs.

Keywords: cell cultures, cytotoxicity, artificial tear, preservatives, buffers, cornea, ocular surface epithelium

1. Introduction

Tear substitutes are widely used in ophthalmology today and are the first-line treatment of multifactorial causes that occur in various cases of irritation of the ocular surface, including dry eye syndrome (DES). Artificial tears contain the following substances as active ingredients: sodium hyaluronate, carbomer, hydroxypropyl methylcellulose (HPMC), carmellose sodium, trehalose, as well as a combination of polyvinyl alcohol and povidone and HPMC together with dextran. In addition to the active ingredient, various preservatives are added to maintain the stability of the drops and suppress microorganism growth: benzalkonium chloride (BAC), cetrimide, cetalkonium chloride, Polyquad®, polyhexanide, and also Oxide®, Purite®, and OcuPure®. Substances that increase the viscosity (prolongators) reduce the rate of removal of the substance from the ocular surface. These include povidone, polyvinyl alcohol, glycerol, propylene glycol, gelatin, methylcellulose, dextran 70, and carboxymethylcellulose. The next component of eye drops is antioxidants; they prevent the decomposition of the active ingredient by atmospheric oxygen. The most commonly used antioxidants are EDTA, bisulfite, thiosulfate, and metabisulfite. Eye drops may contain buffer substances (systems), which allow maintaining the pH of the drug in the range of 6–8. This is necessary to ensure that the pH of the drops is similar to the normal acidity of a human tear (7.14–7.82). With such similarity, the active substances can easily penetrate the cornea into the anterior chamber of the eye, without causing discomfort during instillation. Examples of buffers are citrate, phosphate, borate, and Tris buffers. Another important component of eye drops is osmotic agents: propylene glycol, glycerol, dextrose, and dextran. These substances provide isotonicity of eye drops in relation to the tear film and maintain osmotic pressure at the level of 305 mOsm/L. Isotonic solutions are better absorbed and well tolerated by the patient.

Thus, in addition to the main pharmaceutical ingredient, eye drops contain a number of excipients, some of which can have an adverse effect on the ocular surface, such as preservatives, buffer system components, and antioxidants.

The inclusion of preservatives in the composition of eye drops is necessary to maintain sterility and prevent their bacterial contamination. According to international standards, the addition of preservatives is mandatory in the manufacture of multidose dosage forms for topical use.

The concentration of the latter in the composition of the eye drops is relatively low; however, the cumulative dose over the entire period of use, especially with their frequent and prolonged use, can be quite high. This is especially important to remember in the context of the development of side effects that can be caused by some of the excipients in eye drops, including artificial tears [1, 2]. The preservatives in the composition of eye drops can be divided into three main types: detergents, oxidizers, and ion buffer systems. Detergent-type preservatives have a broad spectrum of antimicrobial action, which makes them quite toxic for corneal and conjunctival cells [3]. Oxidizing preservatives are less toxic than detergents, while they are effective against bacteria even at low concentrations, which minimizes their adverse effects on conjunctival and corneal epithelial cells [4]. The ion buffer preservative with an antibacterial and antifungal effect is similar to oxidizing agents in its mechanism of action [5]. It is less cytotoxic for the cells of the ocular surface than conventional preservatives but is not yet included in the composition of tear substitutes currently [6].

In the United States, many comparative clinical studies have been conducted to assess the efficacy of tear substitutes. In the published report of the Dry Eye Workshop, it was noted that despite the fact that many tear substitutes improved the ocular surface condition, there was no reliable evidence that any of the drugs was superior to another, while the inflammation of the ocular surface could worsen in the presence of preservatives in their composition [7, 8].

Recently, studies of not only developed but already available drugs have been increasingly using in vitro test systems, among which models with monolayer cell cultures are the simplest and most accessible ones [9–11]. Cells grown in vitro retain many metabolic features of the parent host tissues and at the same time lack tissue and organ interrelations and regulatory effects of the nervous and endocrine systems and have very limited compensatory capabilities. These features of cell cultures provide an opportunity to investigate the interaction of chemical agents directly with the cell itself, to identify changes in cellular and subcellular structures that can be masked in whole-organism settings. It is known that cells affected by various biologically active substances can undergo changes in morphology, cell growth rate, time of death, and degree of disintegration; therefore, it is advisable for each dosage form to assess its effect on cell survival [12]. In toxicology studies, various cell cultures are used. They differ in origin, belonging to a particular tissue type, sensitivity to various xenobiotics, as well as in their ability to proliferate. The selection of a test system in each case depends on the purposes and objectives of the study. To assess the safety of ophthalmic drugs, the most informative are test systems based on human eye tissue cells [13–18].

The purpose of this study was to comparatively analyze the cytotoxic effect of 21 tear substitutes on human corneal epithelial cells in vitro.

2. Materials and methods

2.1 Test drugs

The study object was 11 tear substitutes with various systems of preservatives (**Table 1**) and buffer systems (**Table 2**), Systane® Ultra, Artelac® Balance, Optive®, Cationorm®, Vismed® Light, Blink® contacts, Stillavit®, Ophtolique®, Lacrisifi®, Hypromellose®-P, and Slezin®, and 7 preservative-free tear substitutes, Hylabak®, Thealoz®, Thealoz Duo®, Hylo-Comod®, Hyloparin-Comod®, Hylosar-Comod®, and Hylomax-Comod® (**Table 2**).

2.2 Cell cultures used

Cells of the immortalized human corneal epithelial cell (HCE) line were used as a test system. This test system has a higher sensitivity to the action of tear substitutes, compared with a test system based on the permanent human conjunctival cell line (Chang conjunctiva, clone 1-5c-4) [17].

2.3 Study design and methods

The effect of artificial tear eye drops on the viability of human corneal epithelial cells was studied in vitro during culturing the cells in Keratinocyte-SFM growth medium (Gibco, USA) containing the test drugs at a concentration of 10% of the

Chemical glass of preservative	Name of preservative/antioxidant	Trade name of tear substitute
Detergents	BAC, EDTA	Slezin®
	BAC, EDTA	Hypromellose®-P
	BAC, EDTA	Lacrisifi®
	BAC, EDTA	Ophtolique®
	Polyhexanide, EDTA	Vismed® Light
	Polyquad®	Systane® Ultra
	Cetalkonium chloride	Cationorm®
Oxidants	Stabilized oxychloro complex	
	Purite®	Optive®
	OcuPure®	Blink® contacts
	Stabilized chlorite complex	
	Oxide®	Artelac® Balance
Other	EDTA	Stillavit®

Table 1.
The main groups of preservatives/oxidants in the tear substitutes.

Buffer systems	Tear substitutes
Citrate buffer (C)	Hylo-Comod®, Hyloparin-Comod®, Hylomax-Comod®, Hylosar-Comod®
Phosphate buffer (P)	Lacrisifi®
Borate buffer (B)	Systane® Ultra, Blink® contacts, Slezin®
Tris buffer	Cationorm®, Hylabak®, Thealoz®, Thealoz Duo®
Combination of buffers	Optive® (B + C), Vismed® Light (P + C), Stillavit® (B + P)
No buffer	Artelac® Balance, Ophtolique®

Table 2.
Buffer systems in the study of tear substitutes.

medium volume at 37°C in a CO_2 incubator in an 5% CO_2 atmosphere. Cells cultured under standard conditions without the addition of drugs were used as control cells. The concentration of tear substitutes for the experiment was selected on the data of clinical use of the test drugs and our own cytotoxicity studies of artificial tears on cell cultures [17]. Cell viability was assessed by their morphology and functional activity using phase-contrast microscopy (FCM) methods, MTT test, and xCELLigence system.

The morphology of the cells in the course of their culturing with the test drugs was evaluated using an inverted Nikon Eclipse TS100 microscope equipped with a camera. To evaluate the effect of tear substitutes on the metabolic activity of human corneal epithelial cells by MTT method, the cells were inoculated in 96-well plates in 200 μl of the growth medium containing the test drugs and cultured as usual for 2 days. After the culturing period, MTT test was performed. The absorbance of the solutions was measured using Fluorofot Charity analyzer (Russia) at a wavelength of 570 nm and a reference wavelength of 630 nm. Mathematical processing of the data was performed by variation statistics methods using Microsoft Excel 2007. Differences were considered significant at $p < 0.05$.

To evaluate the effect of tear substitutes on the adhesion and proliferative activity of corneal epithelial cells using xCELLigence system, 1×10^4 HCE cells were inoculated per well of the E-plate in 100 μl of the growth medium containing the test drugs. The plates were placed in the real-time cell analyzer dual purpose (RTCA-DP) (ACEA Biosciences), and adhesion and cell proliferation dynamics was monitored in real time for 24 h. The results were analyzed using RTCA Software 1.2.1 (Roche). The change in impedance at microelectrodes due to cell attachment and spreading was expressed as Cell Index; the value of which is automatically calculated by the program: Cell Index = (RnRb)/t, where Rb is the initial impedance value in the well containing the cell growth medium only (negative control) and Rn is the impedance value at any time t in the well containing the test cells (positive control) in addition to the growth medium. The Cell Index thus reflects changes in the number of cells, the quality of cell attachment, and the morphology of the cells in the well, which may vary over time. The data were presented as the mean value (M) ± standard deviation, the significance of differences was calculated by the Mann-Whitney U-test, and differences were considered significant at $p < 0.05$.

3. Results and discussion

3.1 MTT test

The MTT test, commonly known as a screening method for measuring cell survival and included in most protocols of molecular biology and medicine [19], revealed differences in the effect of the test tear substitutes on the metabolic activity of the corneal epithelial cells. The results of the MTT test are presented as a histogram, where the viability of cells cultured in growth media with the addition of eye drops is expressed as a percentage relative to the control (**Figure 1**).

The MTT test showed that the tear substitutes containing preservatives from the group of detergents, especially BAC at various concentrations, have the greatest toxicity to corneal epithelial cells: Lacrisifi® (BAC 0.1 mg/mL), Slezin® (BAC 0.075 mg/mL), Ophtolique® (BAC 0.1 mg/mL), Hypromellose®-P (BAC 0.1 mg/mL), and Cationorm® (cetalkonium chloride). Cell viability in the presence of these drugs was close to zero. The exceptions in this group were Vismed® Light (polyhexanide), which did not have a toxic effect at the studied concentration, and Systane® Ultra (Polyquad®), which had a moderate toxic effect. This was probably due to the fact that Vismed® Light contains the preservative polyhexanide, which is rarely included in the composition of tear substitutes. This preservative has a limited antifungal activity and no irritating effect on the human corneal epithelial cells [5]. The eye drops Systane® Ultra contain Polyquad® (polydronium chloride), which is a detergent-type preservative derived from BAC. It is unique in that bacterial cells attract Polyquad®, while corneal epithelial cells tend to repel it. Despite the occurrence of some superficial epithelial lesions, it is better tolerated than other detergent-type preservative agents [20]. Extremely high toxicity to corneal epithelial cells was also shown by the tear substitutes containing oxidants as preservatives: the stabilized oxychloro complex Optive® (Purite®) and the stabilized chlorite complex Artelac® Balance (Oxide®). The least toxic in this group was the Blink® tear substitute with OcuPure® as a preservative. It is thought that oxidative preservatives have a mild cytotoxic effect and are well tolerated and safe [21]; however, it has been found that this group of preservatives can cause superficial punctate keratitis with prolonged use [22]. The group of tear substitutes consisting of only one drug (Stillavit®), which showed moderate toxicity compared to artificial tears with detergent- and oxidative-type preservatives, includes the antioxidant EDTA (sodium edetate). It is a chelating agent, which, while not being a true preservative, can increase the antimicrobial activity of the main disinfectant while reducing its concentration. It chelates the divalent cations of calcium and magnesium, making the microorganisms more vulnerable to the preservative. Since EDTA chelates calcium and magnesium ions, it can also have a slight toxic effect on the corneal

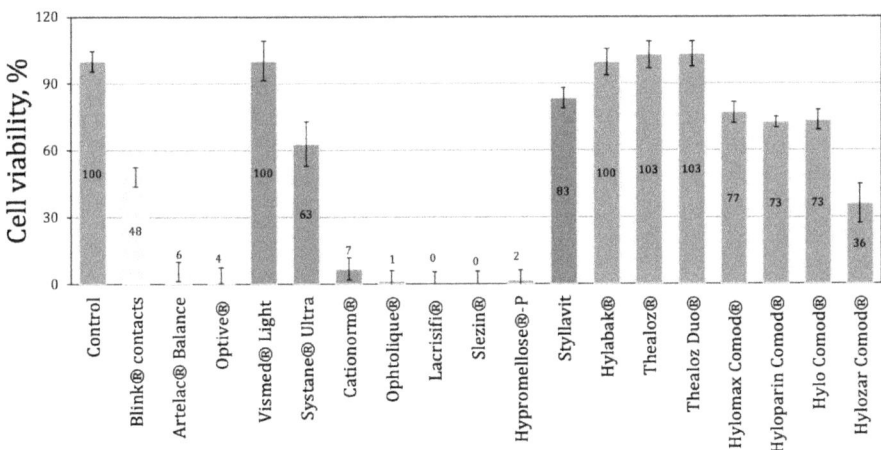

Figure 1.
HCE viability histograms on day 3 of culturing in the medium with a concentration of the test drugs of 10% of the growth medium volume. The drugs were added to the growth medium at the time of inoculating the cells.

cells, which need these ions for metabolism. Although EDTA does not generally have a pronounced toxic effect, there is evidence that patients with severe DES often complain of discomfort after using drugs containing EDTA [23].

The results of the study indicate the cytotoxic effect of tear substitutes with different chemical groups of preservatives on corneal epithelial cells. In scientific literature, this problem is currently covered quite objectively and completely. In addition to the active ingredient, preservatives, and some other excipients, tear substitutes contain various buffer systems (**Table 2**), which can have an adverse effect on corneal and conjunctival epithelial cells. Information on the comparative toxicity of the buffer systems included in the eye drops is almost not available. Nevertheless, separate reports present data on the occurrence of keratopathy and deposition of calcium hydroxyapatite in a transparent layer of the cornea, after using eye drops containing phosphate buffer [24, 25]. Phosphate-containing tear substitutes are widely used in the composition of ophthalmic dosage forms in EU countries, about a third of all buffered drugs contain phosphates as a buffer. The European Committee on Human Medicinal Products (CHMP) gives preference to the use of phosphate-containing drugs, reasoning that the risks do not exceed adverse reactions that occur during their use, since the proportion of complications is less than 1 case per 10,000 sold vials of tear substitutes. Calcification is a multifactorial complication and can occur without the use of phosphate-containing drugs. Preference in selecting phosphate-containing tear substitutes should be given if it is consistent with the low risk of corneal calcification, especially in serious pathology, and on an individual case basis. It is not currently clear what phosphate concentration is critical for the onset of corneal calcification. Quite recently, preference has been given to borate buffers, which possess antimicrobial activity, showed good biocompatibility with the ocular surface both in vivo and in vitro and are considered safer [26, 27]. Tris buffers are also included in some dosage forms and have been found to be effective and low toxic [28].

As our studies have shown, the viability of human corneal epithelial cells depends, among other things, on the composition of the buffer system used in tear substitutes containing no preservatives. The lowest metabolic activity of cells in the study of a line of preservative-free tear substitutes was observed in the presence of Hylosar-Comod® containing citrate buffer together with dexpanthenol. The pronounced cytotoxic effect of Hylosar-Comod® on corneal epithelial cells can be due to the sensitivity of this test system to the combination of the drug ingredients. This question requires further investigation. A higher level of metabolism in cells was detected in the presence of three preservative-free tear substitutes containing citrate buffer (Hylomax-Comod®, Hyloparin-Comod®, and Hylo-Comod®). The average level of cell viability in this case ranged from 73 to 77%. The preservative-free tear substitutes Hylabak®, Thealoz®, and Thealoz Duo® with Tris buffer showed no toxicity to corneal epithelial cells in our studies (**Figure 1**).

3.2 xCELLigence analysis

Based on the data obtained in the MTT test, eight products with various types of preservatives were selected from a wide range of tear substitutes for xCELLigence analysis: Artelac® and Blink® (oxidants), Ophtolique® and Systane® Ultra (detergents), Stillavit® (EDTA), Hylo-Comod®, Thealoz Duo®, and Hylosar-Comod® (preservative free). These drugs within their groups showed varying degrees of toxicity to the metabolic activity of corneal epithelial cells. The xCELLigence real-time cell analyzer (RTCA) technology is based on the use of microelectronic cell sensors integrated into the bottom of the wells of special culture plates (E-Plate). The resistance measured between the electrodes in a separate well depends on the geometry of the electrode, the concentration of ions in the well, and whether the cells are attached to the electrodes. In the absence of cells, the electrode resistance is mainly determined by the ionic environment both at the electrode/solution interface and in the entire volume. The cells attached to the electrode surfaces act as insulators and thus change the local ionic medium at the electrode/solution interface, which will increase the resistance. Thus, the more cells spread on the electrodes, the higher the resistance of the electrodes. The presence of cells on the electrodes in the wells of the E-Plate affects the local state of the ionic environment, which leads to a change in the resistance on the electrodes. The Cell Index value is an indicator of electrical potential, which reflects the cell status. The Cell Index can be used for real-time monitoring of cell viability: their morphology, degree of adhesion, cell growth (proliferation) dynamics, and other important parameters [12]. Continuous monitoring of the effect of tear substitutes on the HCE cell line in real time using the xCELLigence system revealed that the studied drugs at a concentration of 10% of the growth medium volume manifested varying degrees of toxicity to the cultured cells. In the course of monitoring, Cell Index-cell cultivation time plots were obtained, that made it possible to assess the cell viability by the degree of their spreading and proliferative activity (**Figure 2**).

As can be seen from the plots, of all the drugs tested using the xCELLigence system, the tear substitute Ophtolique® with BAC has the highest toxicity to the corneal epithelial cells (**Figure 2B**). The Cell Index equal to zero throughout the observation period indicates that cell adhesion has never occurred. In the presence of Artelac® Balance (**Figure 2A**) containing the preservative Oxide®, adhesion occurs within 1 h, but after 5 h, the cells begin to detach from the bottom of the wells, and after 10 h, no viable cells were detected. The xCELLigence analysis revealed an adverse effect of preservative-free Hylosar-Comod® containing citrate buffer with dexpanthenol on the cell culture (**Figure 2D**). This drug turned out to be the most toxic drug from the group of preservative-free tear substitutes; its cytotoxic effect was comparable to that of Blink® containing an oxidative-type preservative (**Figure 2A**). In the presence of these drugs, the cells could only adhere and spread. In the presence of Hylo-Comod® (**Figure 2D**) and Systane® Ultra (**Figure 2B**), the corneal epithelial cells adhered and spread, but their proliferation dynamics was low. Cell proliferation in the presence of Stillavit® (**Figure 2C**) was slightly lower than in the control, and the presence of Thealoz Duo® (**Figure 2D**) was comparable to the control, indicating that Stillavit® was moderately toxic and Thealoz Duo® did not exhibit toxicity at the given concentration to corneal epithelial cells.

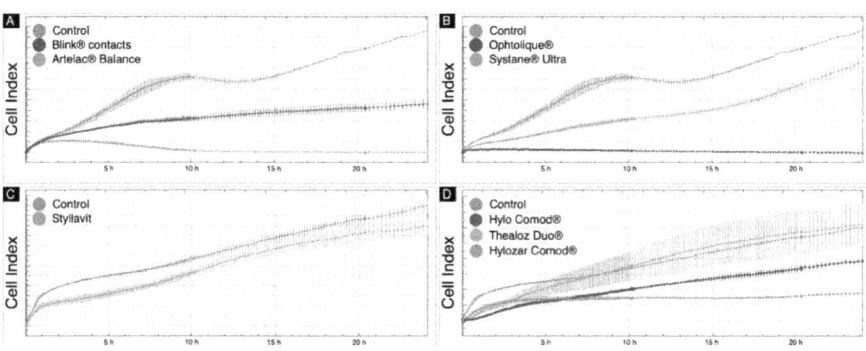

Figure 2.
Monitoring of the effect of tear substitutes with various types of preservatives ((A) oxidants, (B) detergents, (C) EDTA, (D) preservative-free drugs) on the viability of HCE cells in real time (proliferation curves). xCELLigence cell analysis.

3.3 Observation of the cells morphology

The results of observation of the HCE cell morphology during their culturing in media containing 10% PCTs with various preservative systems are shown in **Figure 3**. In the pictures presented, the human corneal cells in the control are well spread, have a typical epithelium-like morphology, and have formed a confluent monolayer on cultivation day 3 (**Figure 3E**).

The morphology of the cells in the presence of the tear substitute Thealoz Duo® is comparable to the control. A slightly less dense monolayer than in the control is formed by the cells in the presence of Stillavit® in the growth medium. With Hylo-Comod®, the monolayer of cells is less dense than in the presence of Thealoz Duo® and Stillavit®. Most of the cells in the presence of the former drug are well spread, but their cytoplasm has a granular structure; a lot of unattached cells are observed. In the presence of the tear substitutes Blink® and Systane® Ultra, the monolayer is formed by about 50%; the cells have a vacuolated granular cytoplasm, which indicates their supressed state. With Hylosar-Comod®, a part of the cells have adhered, and intercellular contacts are found between them; in the presence of Artelac®, only single adherent cells are detected, and in the presence of Ophtolique®, no spread cells are found at all; most of the cells have a rounded shape. The cell structure is granular, with vacuoles; invagination of the cytoplasmic membrane is observed. Many cellular fragments are found in the growth medium. These observations suggest a launch of cell death processes. Thus, the results of the MTT test are consistent with the results of the xCELLigence cell analysis and the cell morphology analysis using phase-contrast microscopy methods.

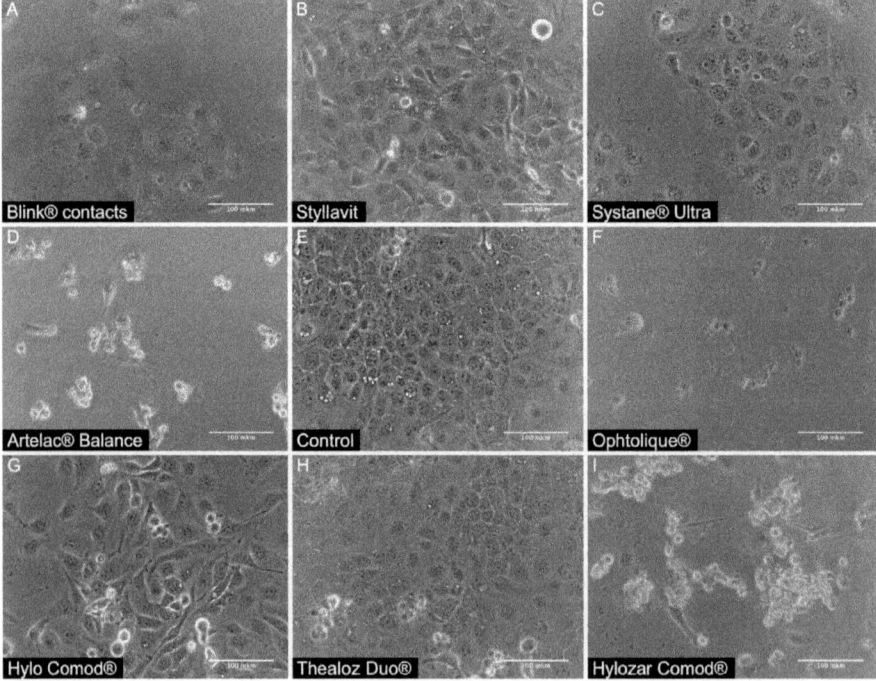

Figure 3.
Morphology of HCE cell line on the third day of culturing in a growth medium containing 10% of the test PCTs with various types of preservatives: oxidants (A, D), detergents (C, F), EDTA (B), and preservative-free drugs (G, H, I). Scale ruler 100 nm (20×). Phase-contrast microscopy.

4. Conclusion

A large number of artificial tears are currently available in the pharmaceutical market. Selecting the right drug for the patient remains a challenge for both the doctor and the patient. This study presents the results of assessing the cytotoxicity of tear substitutes, which demonstrate that these drugs can have a cytostatic effect in vitro and differ in their cytotoxic potential. Comparing the cytotoxicity of artificial tears is necessary for the rational selection of a drug that promotes maximum clinical efficacy and a higher safety profile. The tear substitutes Hylabak®, Thealoz®, and Thealoz Duo® that do not contain preservatives in their composition had not cytotoxic effect on the cells. Vismed® Light containing the preservative polyhexanide was not toxic, either. It was found that the so-called mild preservatives can also have an adverse effect on the ocular surface. Among the artificial tears, the greatest toxic effect on corneal epithelial cells was observed in the tear substitutes Ophtolique®, Lacrisifi®, Hypromellose®, Slezin®, and Cationorm® containing BAC at various concentrations as preservative and in the artificial tears Artelac® Balance (Purite®) and Optive® (Oxide®). The study showed the possibility in principle to use in vitro systems for the comparative assessment of the cytotoxic effect of tear substitutes. It should be noted, however, that the test system under consideration has a number of limitations due to the very nature of the method. In particular, studies on cell cultures cannot take into account such aspects that are important in terms of general toxicology as the route of delivery of a chemical agent into the body, its distribution, elimination, and other toxicodynamics issues. Like with the use of other model test systems, extrapolation of the results obtained to the whole body requires great caution, especially when it comes to quantitative indicators. However, in vitro testing provides information on the potential effects of drugs and their specific effects. Given that the problem of drug therapy of patients with DES has been recently attracting increasing attention of ophthalmologists due to both the increasing prevalence of DES and the increasing range of "artificial tear" drugs, screening the cytotoxicity of a wide range of tear substitutes using test systems based on cell cultures can promote the rational selection of these drugs.

Conflict of interest

The author declares no competing interests.

Author details

Olga I. Aleksandrova[1*], Igor N. Okolov[2], Julia I. Khorolskaya[1], Natalia A. Mikhailova[1], Diana M. Darvish[1] and Miralda I. Blinova[1]

1 Institute of Cytology of the Russian Academy of Science, Saint Petersburg, Russia

2 Sv. Fyodorov Eye Microsurgery Federal State Institution, Saint-Petersburg, Russia

*Address all correspondence to: elga.aleks@gmail.com

IntechOpen

© 2019 The Author(s). Licensee IntechOpen. This chapter is distributed under the terms of the Creative Commons Attribution License (http://creativecommons.org/licenses/by/3.0), which permits unrestricted use, distribution, and reproduction in any medium, provided the original work is properly cited. (cc) BY

References

[1] Baudouin C, Labbe A, Liang H, Pauly A, Brignole-Baudouin F. Preservatives in eye drops: The good, the bad and the ugly. Progress in Retinal and Eye Research. 2010;9:312-334. DOI: 10.1016/j.preteyeres.2010.03.001

[2] Whitson J, Petroll W. Corneal epithelial cell viability following exposure to ophthalmic solutions containing preservatives and/or antihypertensive agents. Advances in Therapy. 2012;29:874-888. DOI: 10.1007/s12325-012-0057-1

[3] Tu E. Balancing antimicrobial efficacy and toxicity of currently available topical ophthalmic preservatives. Saudi Journal of Ophthalmology. 2014;28(3):182-187. DOI: 10.1016/j.sjopt.2014.06.006

[4] Elder D, Crowley P. Antimicrobial preservatives part one: Choosing a preservative system. American Pharmaceutical Review. 2012. Available from: http://www.americanpharmaceuticalreview.com/Featured-Articles/38886-Antimicrobial-Preservatives-Part-One-Choosing-a-Preservative-System/

[5] Freeman P, Kahook M. Preservatives in topical ophthalmic medications: Historical and clinical perspectives. Expert Review of Ophthalmology. 2009;4(1):59-64

[6] Ammar D, Noecker R, Kahook M. Effects of benzalkonium chloride-preserved, polyquad-preserved, and sofZia-preserved topical glaucoma medications on human ocular epithelial cells. Advances in Therapy. 2010;27(11):837-845. DOI: 10.1007/s12325-010-0070-1

[7] Schiffman R, Christianson M, Jacobsen G, Hirsch J, Reis B. Reliability and validity of the ocular surface disease index. Archives of Ophthalmology. 2000;118:615-621

[8] Management and therapy of dry eye disease: Report of the management and therapy Subcommittee of the International Dry Eye WorkShop (2007). The Ocular Surface. 2007;5(2):163-178

[9] Danchenko EO. Evaluation of cytotoxicity of pharmaceutical substances using cell cultures. Immunopathology, allergology, infectology=Immunopatologija, Allergologija, Infektologija. 2012;2: 22-31. (In Russ.)

[10] Eropkin MJ, Eropkina EM. The Cell Cultures as a Model System Toxicity Studies and Screening of Cytoprotective Drugs. SPb.: Morsar AV; 2003 (in Russ.)

[11] Anikina LV, Puhov SA, Dubrovskaja ES, Afanas'eva SV, Klochkov SG. Comparative determination of cell viability using the MTT and Resazurin. Fundamental Research = Fundamental'nye issledovaniya. 2014;12:1423-1427. (In Russ.)

[12] Urcan E, Haertel U, Styllou M, Hickel R, Scherthan H, Reichl F. Real-time xCELLigence impedance analysis of the cytotoxicity of dental composite components on human gingival fibroblasts. Dental Materials. 2010;26(1):51-58. DOI: 10.1016/j.dental.2009.08.007

[13] Aleksandrova OI, Okolov IN, Takhtaev YV, Khorolskaya YI, Khintuba TS, Blinova MI. Comparative evaluation of the cytotoxicity of antimicrobial eye drops. Ophthalmological Bulletin. 2015;8(1):89-97. (In Russ.)

[14] Aleksandrova OI, Khorolskaya YI, Maychuk DY, Blinova MI. A study of the overall cytotoxicity of aminoglycoside and fluoroquinolone antibiotics on

cell cultures. Ophthalmology Bulletin. 2015;5:39-48. (In Russ.)

[15] Aleksandrova OI, Okolov IN, Khorolskaya YI, Blinova MI, Churakov TK. Evaluation of the effect of benzalkonium chloride on the cytotoxicity of Nettacin and Tobrex eye drops in vitro. Modern Technologies in Ophthalmology. 2016;3:163-166. (In Russ.)

[16] Aleksandrova OI, Okolov IN, Khorolskaya YI, Panova IE, Blinova MI. Possibilities of cellular technologies for rational pharmacotherapy of ocular pathologies. Modern Technologies in Ophthalmology. 2017;7:5-7. (In Russ.)

[17] Aleksandrova OI, Okolov IN, Khorolskaya YI, Panova IE, Blinova MI. Evaluation of cytotoxicity of tear substitutes using an in vitro system. Ophthalmology. 2017;14(1):59-64. DOI: 10.18008/1816-5095-2017-1-59-66. (In Russ.)

[18] Aleksandrova OI, Okolov IN, Khorolskaya YI, Panova IE, Blinova MI. The effect of non-steroidal anti-inflammatory eye drops on corneal and conjunctival epithelial cells in vitro. Ophthalmology. 2017;15(3):251-259. DOI: 10.18008/1816-5095-2017-3-251-259. (In Russ.)

[19] Langdon SP, editor. Cancer Cell Culture: Methods and Protocols. Ser. Methods in Molecular Medicine. Vol. 88. Totowa, NJ: Humana Press; 2003. p. 165-169

[20] Epstein S, Ahdoot M, Marcus E, Asbell P. Comparative toxicity of preservatives on immortalized corneal and conjunctival epithelial cells. Journal of Ocular Pharmacology and Therapeutics. 2009;25(2):113-119

[21] Noecker R. Effects of common ophthalmic preservatives on ocular health. Advances in Therapy. 2001;18(5):205-215

[22] Schrage N, Frentz M, Spoeler F. The ex vivo eye irritation test (EVEIT) in evaluation of artificial tears: Purite-preserved versus unpreserved eye drops. Graefe's Archive for Clinical and Experimental Ophthalmology. 2012;250(9):1333-1340. DOI: 10.1007/s00417-012-1999-3

[23] Samar K. Basak preservatives and ocular surface diseases. Kerala Journal of Ophthalmology. 2016;18(4):311-316

[24] Schrage N, Frentz M, Reim M. Changing the composition of buffered eye-drops prevents undesired side effects. The British Journal of Ophthalmology. 2010;94:1519-1522. DOI: 10.1136/bjo.2009.177386

[25] Mueller-Lierheim W. Traenenersatz- und Kontaktlinsenbenetzungsloesungen. In: Köln Biermann, editor. Aktuelle Kontaktologie; 2015. 8-15

[26] Houlsby R, Ghajar M, Chavez G. Antimicrobial activity of borate-buffered solutions. Antimicrobial Agents and Chemotherapy. 1986;29:803-806

[27] Lehmann D, Cavet M, Richardson M. Nonclinical safety evaluation of boric acid and a novel borate-buffered contact lens multi-purpose solution, Biotrue™ multi-purpose solution. Contact Lens & Anterior Eye. 2010;33(Suppl 1):S24-S32. DOI: 10.1016/j.clae.2010.06.010

[28] Graupner O, Hausmann C. The alternation of the pH in the anterior chamber of the rabbits eye burned with smallest volumes of high concentrated acid and base [in German]. Albrecht von Graefes Archiv für Klinische und Experimentelle Ophthalmologie. 1968;176:48-53

Chapter 2

Study of the Cytotoxic Activity of Haarlem Oil on Different Cell Lines and a Higher Organism, *Steinernema feltiae*

Khairan Khairan, Torsten Burkholz, Mareike Kelkel, Vincent Jamier, Karl-Herbert Schäfer and Claus Jacob

Abstract

Haarlem oil (HO) is a semisynthetic product made by combining terpene oil and sulfur atoms at high temperatures. HO contains organosulfur compounds; these compounds are known to have strong antioxidant properties, such as superoxide dismutase (SOD). This study provides a brief overview of the effects of HO cytotoxicity on several cell lines using several cytotoxicity test methods. The crystal violet (CV) staining assay showed that HO had a strong toxic effect on the A549 cell line. The test results of the trypan blue and celltiter-Glo assay methods showed that HO has a strong cytotoxic effect on HL-60 cells. The results of the MTT and XTT assays indicated that HO produced a fairly strong toxic effect on HL-60 cells and U937 cells. A hoechst staining assay showed that HO was able to increase (induce) apoptotic cell levels and reduce mitotic cell levels after 24 hours of incubation. However, in this study, we were not able to detect any effect of HO on activation and inhibition of the K562 cell line through the NF-κB pathway. Meanwhile, the live and dead assay showed that HO tends to cause apoptosis. The nematicidal assay showed that HO showed moderate activity against *Steinernema feltiae*.

Keywords: Haarlem oil, cytotoxicity activity, organosulfur compounds, *Steinernema feltiae*

1. Introduction

Haarlem oil (HO) was first introduced in the Netherlands by Thomas Monsieur, a French scientist, as a dietary supplement and stamina aid. In the sixteenth century, a Dutch researcher named Claas Tilly used HO for the first time for the treatment of kidney and urinary stones. HO became increasingly popular in the Netherlands as a health product (**Figure 1**). HO production at that time continued to increase, eventually attracting the attention of scientists because of its efficacy and usefulness in the fields of health and beauty. In the nineteenth century, HO's effects and uses started to be studied pharmacologically. In 1924, HO was widely traded in France as a food supplement. In the 1980s and 1990s, HO again received the attention of scientists because of its sulfur content. At present, HO is produced semi-synthetically from natural products, including terpene oil and sulfur elements, which are combined at high temperatures. Research shows that, in addition to sulfur compounds, HO also contains iminosugars. Iminosugars are compounds containing nitrogen atom bases in their endocyclic structure. It is known that this nitrogen atom is partially responsible for HO's activity. A study of the literature also shows that HO contains polyunsaturated essential oils; polyunsaturated essential oils are known to have strong antioxidant effects, such as in superoxide dismutase (SOD) [1–3].

HO has been reported to be effective in treating rheumatic diseases, bronchitis, and diseases of the liver and kidneys [2, 3]. Histological and bio-clinical tests on mice showed that the sulfo-terpene in HO stimulated the adrenal cortex by causing mice to secrete adrenocorticotropic hormone (ACTH) and eliminating corticosteroids in urine [4]. HO also has strong antiseptic properties, which are thought to originate from its terpene content. Other studies have shown that, when applied to bronchial-pulmonary tissue for 15–60 minutes, HO anti-inflammatory action and increased the action of SOD by increasing the levels of thiol (–SH) group in plasma. Antioxidant activity tests have shown that HO is able to increase SOD enzyme activity. Toxicology and posology tests showed no cases of intoxication in patients given HO at a dose of 2500 mg/kg [5]. X-ray analysis of bronchitis patients treated with HO at a dose of 10 mg/kg for 10 days showed improvements [6].

In the body, sulfur is essential because it functions as a regulatory agent in bile glands, as a stimulator in the respiratory system, and as a toxin neutralizer, and also plays a role in the allergic response. In cells, sulfur plays a role in the synthesis of proteins and also contributes to the synthesis of essential amino acids (such as cysteine and methionine), vitamins (thiamine or vitamin B_1, Biotin, and B_6), and coenzyme A (CoA), which plays a role in many metabolic processes. Sulfur compounds also play a major role in the prevention of various cancers and infection by microorganisms such as bacteria and fungi.

HO is a natural product containing unusual sulfur compounds, such as thiosulfinate, polysulphane, 1,2-dithiin, and 1,2-dithiole-3-thione. HO also contains several other isothiocyanates. These compounds are also found in many other natural ingredients such as onions (*Allium* sp.), mustard, and asparagus. Unusual sulfur compounds generally contain reactive sulfur species (RSS), which function as antioxidants and have cytotoxic activities, which give them their anticancer, antibacterial, antifungal, and antisclerodermal effects [7]. This study presents a brief overview of the effects of HO cytotoxicity on several cell lines, using several cytotoxicity test methods such as Crystal Violet (CV), CellTiter-Glo, Trypan Blue, MTT, XTT, NF-κB pathway, Hoechst staining, and Live and Dead assays. This article also provides brief information about HO activity against *Steinernema feltiae* (*S. feltiae*). *S. feltiae* is a microscopic entomopathogenic nematode. This means that

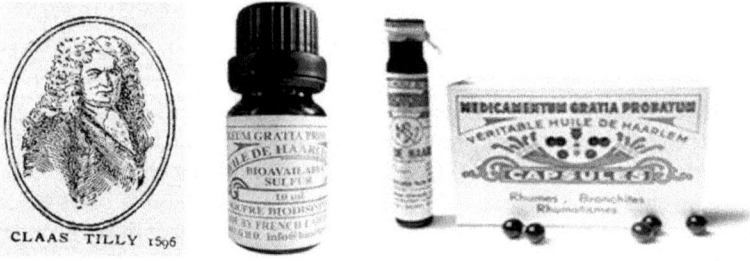

Figure 1.
Products of Haarlem oil.

it is itself a parasite in other parasites, especially insects and their eggs [8]. *S. feltiae* was selected as a test organism is because this organism is a complex organism and can be used as a model for whole organisms [9, 10].

2. Cytotoxicity studies of Haarlem oil study cytotoxicity by crystal violet staining assay

Crystal violet (CV), or Tris(4-(dimethylamino)phenyl)methylium chloride, is a triarylmethane dye which is used to investigate cell viability responses. CV staining is used mainly in living cell membranes, because this dye is able to bind to proteins and DNA in cells. Cells that die will lose adherence and then disappear from the cell population. Losses from the population of cells reduce the amount of dye staining in a culture, which enables the researcher to count the number of cells in a monolayer culture via absorption of dye by the cells. This test is a simple, fast method of cell viability screening and is useful for acquiring information about relative cell density. CV can also be used to measure the cytotoxicity of a compound [11, 12].

The CV test has major advantages over other cytotoxic tests: in a CV test, after staining, changes in cell morphology can be observed and stored for a long time. At present, research on the effects of HO cytotoxicity is still limited. Therefore, this article provides a brief overview of the effects of HO cytotoxicity on several cell lines such as 3T3, CT26, HT29, A549, HUVEC, MCF7, HepG2, and OVCAR cell lines.

At present, HO is sold as a supplement for maintaining stamina and as an antioxidant. HO has been studied previously because of its organosulfur compound content, which may have potential for medical treatments. The mechanism of HO activity against cells is not yet fully understood. Knowledge of the biological activity of HO, especially as related to the behavior of redox-modulators, is also still very limited [1, 12].

In this study, the results of HO cytotoxicity on several cells are expressed in percentages of cell viability, by measuring the Optical Density (OD) of cells at a wavelength of 590 nm (OD_{590}). OD indicates the absorbance of a sample measured at a specific wavelength, and is a common method used to measure concentration, growth conditions, and cell reproduction abilities.

To determine the cytotoxicity of HO, we used several levels of HO concentration, from 13.125 to 50 ppm. In this test, we used a 0.1% cytotoxic agent solution of detergent Nonylphenoxypolyethoxy ethanol (NP40). This detergent acts to break down and open membranes in cells, including the membrane's core. **Figure 1** shows HO's effect on 3T3, CT26, HT29, A549, HUVEC, MCF7, HepG2, and OVCAR cell lines at various concentrations.

The results show that HO has almost the same toxic effect as NP40. In the OVCAR cell line, HO had the highest toxic effect after 72 hours of incubation, while for the HT29 cell line, HO had a very small effect. HO had relatively similar cytotoxic effects on the 3T3, CT26, A549, HUVEC, MCF7, and HepG2 cell lines (**Figure 2**).

EC_{50} (half maximal effective concentration) is the concentration of a drug, compound, antibody, or toxicant capable of inhibiting growth by 50% after exposure for a certain amount of time. The EC_{50} value of HO on several cell lines was determined using OriginPro 7.5 software. The EC_{50} values of HO obtained from the CV staining assay method can be seen in **Table 1**. **Table 1** shows that HO had the most active toxic effect on A549 cell lines (adenocarcinomic human alveolar basal epithelial cells), with an EC_{50} value of 6.30 ppm. In addition, HO also showed a strong cytotoxic effect on CT26 and HepG2 cell lines, with EC_{50} values of 6.49 and 6.50, respectively. Meanwhile, HO showed EC50 values of 15.19 and 15.20 ppm, respectively, on the HUVEC and 3T3 cell lines [13].

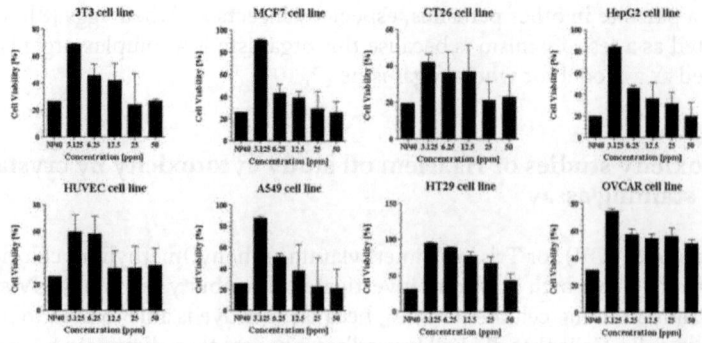

Figure 2.
The percentage of cell viabilities of 3T3, CT26, HT29, A549, HUVEC, MCF7, HepG2 and OVCAR cell lines after been exposed to HO for 72 hours by CV staining assay. Data are expressed as the percentage of viability % ± SD.

Cell line	Characteristics	EC_{50} value [ppm]
3T3	Fibroblast cell line	15.19
HUVEC	Human umbilical vein endothelial cells line	15.20
CT26	Colon carcinoma cell line	6.49
HT29	Human colon carcinoma cells line	>50.0
MCF7	Breast cancer cell line	6.50
A549	Adeno carcinomic human alveolar basal epithelial cells line	6.30
HepG2	Perpetual liver tissue cell line	6.50
OVCAR	Human epithelial carcinoma of the ovary cell line	9.07

Table 1.
The characteristics and EC_{50} values of HO on several cell lines were tested with a CV staining assay.

2.1 Study cytotoxicity on HL-60 cell line

The CellTiter-Glo luminescent cell viability assay is a homogeneous method used to determine the number of active cells in cell cultures. This method quantifies cells based on the presence of adenosine triphosphate (ATP) nucleotides in cells. In this method, the presence of ATP is interpreted as an indicator of cell proliferation and an indicator of energy changes in the cell's biological system. ATP is commonly found in living cells because it plays a role in catabolic and anabolic cell processes. The measurement of ATP is fundamental in the study of cells, as the quantities of ATP directly correlate with cell populations [14]. This method uses the enzyme luciferase, which uses ATP to produce luminescence. This luminescence is then measured by the amount of light, or signal, produced, which is strongly correlated to the amount of ATP in the cell population. ATP quantities are highly correlated with the number of living cells [14].

In this method, the test compounds are diluted at certain concentrations and incubated for 8, 24, and 48 hours. The amount of ATP is measured at the end of the incubation time. The results showed that, at a concentration of 1:10, HO was able to reduce ATP in HL-60 cells by 50%, while at a concentration of 1:5, HO was unable to reduce ATP, because the cells were lysed or killed due to a decrease in cell glycogenesis. Glycogenesis is crucial for the formation of ATP; and the decrease in glycogenesis results in the halt of glycogen formation, leading to cell death. The results also showed that HO was able to reduce the ATP in HL-60 cells at all incubation times [15]. This shows that the reduction in ATP by HO occurs very quickly (**Figure 3**).

Trypan Blue assay is a method used to determine the viability of a cell. The basic principle of this method is that normal cells have intact cell membranes that are able to bind to foreign substances, such as the Trypan Blue dye. In abnormal cells, however, the cell membrane does not have the ability to bind foreign substances onto the cell [16]. In this test, a cell suspension is mixed with Trypan Blue dye, then the cell is observed visually and the viability is calculated using a microscope. Observations were made by examining whether these cells would repel or uptake the dye. In this test, viable cells exhibit clear cytoplasm because their cell membranes cannot be penetrated by the dye, while nonviable cells show blue cytoplasm, because damage to the cell membranes allow them to be easily penetrated by foreign substances such as Trypan Blue. The results showed that HO had a significant cytotoxic effect on cells at all treatment durations and concentrations used. These results also showed that HO at high concentrations (i.e., HO: MilliQ water (1:5) and (1:1)) had a strong effect on the percentage of viability of HL-60 cells, with a percent viability of <10% after 8 hours of incubation. If the incubation time is further extended to 24 and 48 hours, the viability decreases to nearly 0% [15]. These results indicate that, out of all the cells tested, HO had the strongest cytotoxic effect on HL-60 cells (**Figure 3**).

The MTT test is a colorimetric, enzyme-based method commonly used to test mitochondrial dehydrogenase activity in cells. This method is frequently used because it is easy, safe, and has a high sensitivity. It is the most commonly used method for testing cell toxicity and viability [17]. The MTT test is used to evaluate the ability of cells to reduce tetrazolium salt or 3-(4, 5-dimethylthiazole-2-yl) 2, 5 diphenyltetrazolium bromide to form insoluble formazan violet crystals. Colored tetrazolium salt, when interacting with cells, will turn purple (formazan). This color is caused by cells undergoing metabolic reduction by the enzyme

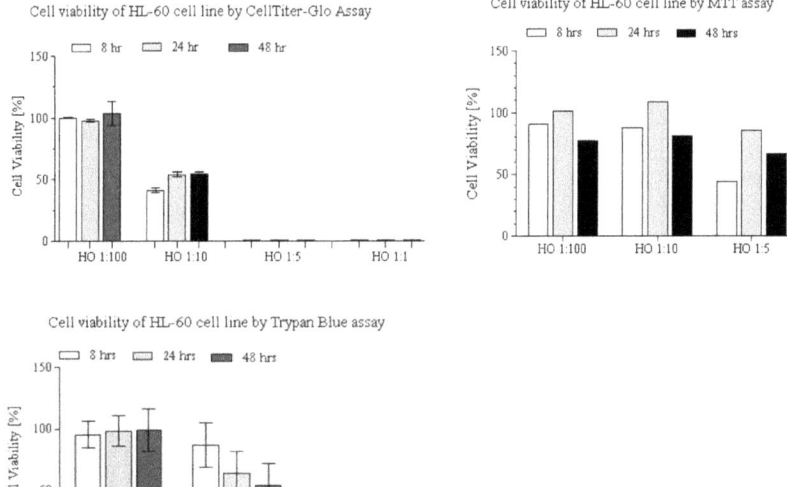

Figure 3.
The cytotoxicity effect of HO on HL-60 cell line using several cytotoxicity assays. Data are expressed as the percentage of viability % ± SD.

dehydrogenase to form NADH or NADPH. It is the absorbance value of this purple color that is measured. This absorbance value is used to determine the cell viability. If the absorbance value observed is smaller than the absorbance value of the control, the cell is undergoing reduction; in other words the cell's ability to proliferate is low. However, on the contrary, if the absorbance produced is higher than the control, the cell's ability to proliferate is very high. If the level of proliferation is too high, however, this can result in cell death, due to potential changes in cell morphology.

This test uses HL-60 cells, which are commonly used as models to study the differentiation of myeloid cells in humans [18, 19]. HL-60 cells exposed to HO at concentrations of 1:100, 1:10, and 1:5 with incubation times of 8, 24, and 48 hours are presented in **Figure 3**. The results indicate that, at a concentration of 1:5, HO was effective at all incubation times, with the percentage of cell viability between 40 and 65%. This means that only 40–65% of cells were able to proliferate. However, at HO concentrations of 1:100 and 1:5, the results were effectively identical, with the percentage of cell viability ranging from 70 to 85% [15] (**Figure 3**).

2.2 Study cytotoxicity on U-973 cell line

In this section, we tried to determine HO's cytotoxicity on the U-937 cell line using the XTT and Hoechst staining assay methods, as well as testing HO's activation and inhibition of U-937 cells through the NF-κB pathway. U937 cells are human histiocytic lymphoma cells. The principle of the XTT test is the breakdown of the tetrazolium salt into formazan by succinate-tetrazolium reductase in the mitochondria, involving electron transfer by mitochondrial and non-mitochondrial enzymes. Compared to MTT, the XTT test is faster, more reproducible, and gives more sensitive results. The viable cells in the XTT test were measured based on the activity of mitochondrial enzymes in reducing tetrazolium salt [20]. In this test, the U-937 cell line was treated with HO for 6, 24, 48, and 72 hours. 24 hours after the HO treatment, the cells were then treated with XTT for 3 hours (6 hours treatment) or 4 hours (24, 48, and 72 hours treatment) and measured with a plate reader at a

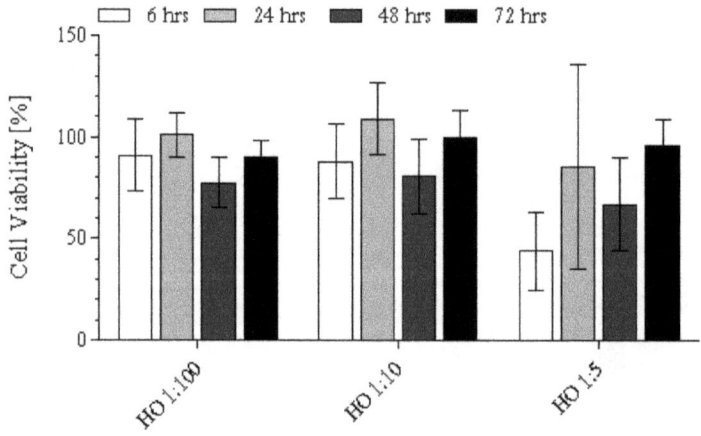

Figure 4.
U937 cell lines were treated with HO using XTT assays. Data are expressed as the percentage of viability % ± SD.

wavelength of 490 nm. The results showed that at a concentration of 1:5, HO had a cytotoxic effect on the U937 cell line (**Figure 4**).

Apoptosis is a biological mechanism characterized as "programmed cell death." Apoptosis is used by multicellular organisms to remove cells that are not needed by the body. Apoptosis shows distinctive morphological features, such as plasma membrane blebbing, cell shrinkage, chromatin condensation, and DNA fragmentation. Mitosis is the process of cell division that identically divides genomes into two daughter cells. Mitosis is generally followed by cytokinesis, which divides the cytoplasm and cell membrane. This process produces two identical daughter cells, which have almost the same distribution of organelles and cell components. Mitosis and cytokinesis make up the mitotic phase (M phase) in the cell cycle, where the initial cell is divided into two daughter cells that have the same genetic origin as the initial cell [21]. In testing HO's effect on U-973 cells, the percentage of apoptotic and mitotic cells was quantified as a fraction. The nuclei of apoptotic cells were observed under a fluorescent microscope using a specific dye, in this case, Hoechst stain 33,342 (Sigma, Bornem, Belgium). The fraction of cells undergoing apoptosis were calculated (at least 300 cells).

Figure 5 shows the ratio of apoptotic and mitotic cells in the U-973 cell line after treatment with HO at a concentration of 1:10. After each treatment, Hoechst staining was performed for 15 minutes and apoptotic and mitotic cells were counted with the fluorescent microscope. The results showed that HO increased the number of apoptotic cells and reduced the number of mitotic cells after 24 hours of incubation (**Figure 5**). The Hoechst staining assay is one method to identify cell apoptosis through cell cycle analysis, mainly sub G1 phase cells.

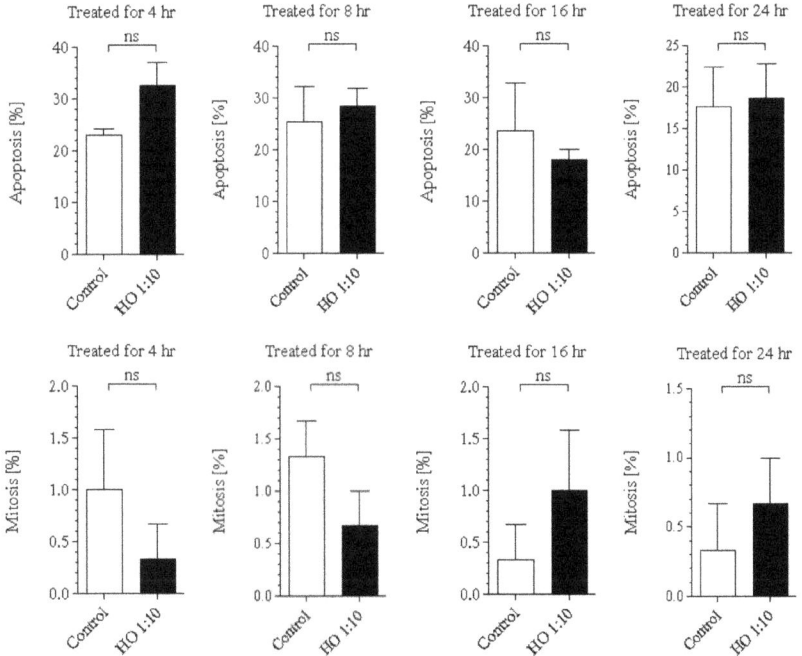

Figure 5.
The U-937 cell line was treated for 4, 8, 16, and 24 hours with HO at a concentration of 1:10. After each treatment, Hoechst staining was performed for 15 minutes. Apoptotic and mitotic cells were counted with the fluorescent microscope, n = 4. Significances are expressed against the control. Data are presented as viability % ± SD. Significances: ns = $p \geq 0.05$, * = $p < 0.05$, ** = $p < 0.01$ and *** = $p < 0.001$.

2.3 Study cytotoxicity on K562 cell lines

NF-κB, or nuclear factor kappa-light-chain enhancer of activated B cells, is a protein complex that controls the DNA transcription process. NF-κB is an important regulator in determining the fate of a cell, such as apoptosis (programmed cell death), control of cell proliferation, and tumorigenesis. The NF-κB pathway is activated by cell exposure to lipopolysaccharide (LPS), inflammatory cytokines such as TNF (Tumor Necrosis Factor) or IL-1 (Interleukin-1), growth factors, lymphokines, oxidant-free radicals, inhaled particles, viral infection, or expression of certain viral or bacterial gene products, UV irradiation, B or T cell activation, and other physiological and non- physiological stimuli. The best NF-κB activators are proinflammatory cytokines IL-1 and TNF, because they cause phosphorylation of κB on the N-terminus domain side. TNF is an excellent activator for binding to TRADD (TNF-Associated Receptor DEATH Domain Protein) receptors and proteins. TRADD binds TRAF2 (TNF Receptor-Associated Factor-2), which recruits NIK (NF-κB-Inducible Kinase) [22, 23]. In this test, we used TNF to activate NF-κB. The activated NF-κB would then cause the expression of genes that keep cells undergoing proliferation and protect cells from conditions that cause death through apoptosis.

The cell type used in this test was a K562 cell line. K562 cells are human chronic myelogenous leukemia lymphoblastoid cells. The K562 cell line was treated with HO at various concentrations for 2 hours, followed by the addition of 20 ng/ml TNF-α for 6 hours. The experiment was repeated five times. The inhibition of the NF-κB pathway in the K562 cell line was analyzed based on the percentage of luciferase enzyme activity.

The results show no detectable effect of HO on the activation and inhibition of the K562 cell line through the NF-κB pathway. According to Keophiphath,

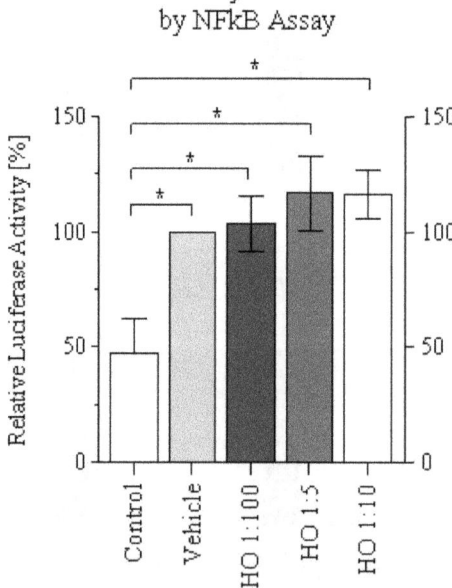

Figure 6.
*The transfected K562 cells were treated with HO with concentrations of: 1:100, 1:10, and 1:5 for 2 hours, followed by a TNF-α-treatment for 6 hours, n = 5. The vehicle was normalized to a cell viability of 100%. Significances are expressed against the control. Data are presented as viability % ± SD. Significances: ns = $p \geq 0.05$, * = $p < 0.05$, ** = $p < 0.01$ and *** = $p < 0.001$.*

a decrease in the synthesis of IL-6 is regulated by the NF-κB pathway; thus, we suspect that this pathway may be involved, but our results were unable to detect any effect of HO on activation and inhibition of the K562 cell line (**Figure 6**).

2.4 Study cytotoxicity on Neuro 2a cell line

In this study, testing on the Neuro 2a cell line was carried out using the Live and Dead assay method. In this method, calcein-AM and propidium iodide are used to determine the viability of Neuro 2a cells, a neuroblastoma-derived cell line (**Figure 7**). There were three reasons for using the Neuro 2a cell line in this study. First, Neuro 2a cells contain GSH at concentrations five times higher than other cell lines, such as PC12 cell line (derived from a transplantable rat pheochromocytoma) [24]. Second, this cell line has expanded to be used as a model to determine the neuronal function of the system. Third, cells from the Neuro 2a cell line are very easy to differentiate using retinoic acid, so that it is structurally close to "real neurons". In this study, the Neuro 2a cell line was used to determine the effect of HO with the presence or absence of Hydrogen peroxide (H_2O_2). Hydrogen peroxide is used to analyze the oxidative effects of stress on compounds [24].

HO activity shows that HO at a concentration of 1:1 with or without H_2O_2 had a moderate toxic effect on Neuro 2a cells, causing a percent viability of about 6%. The morphology of Neuro 2a cell structure after exposure to HO can be seen in **Figure 8**. The results show that Neuro 2a cells tend to experience apoptosis (bubbling) following HO exposure at a concentration of 1:5 after 24 hours incubation.

2.5 Activity on *Steinernema feltiae*

Steinernema feltiae (*S. feltiae*) is an entomopathogenic nematode used as a 'phytoprotectant' due to its consumption of fly eggs and larvae. Because *S. feltiae* is

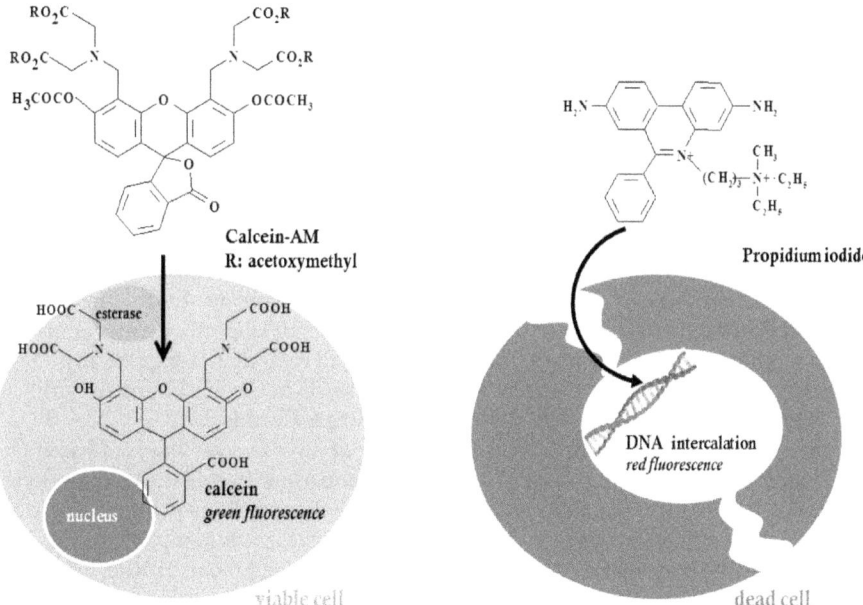

Figure 7.
Schematic representation of a live and dead assay using Calcein-AM and PI staining to determine viable and dead cells [25].

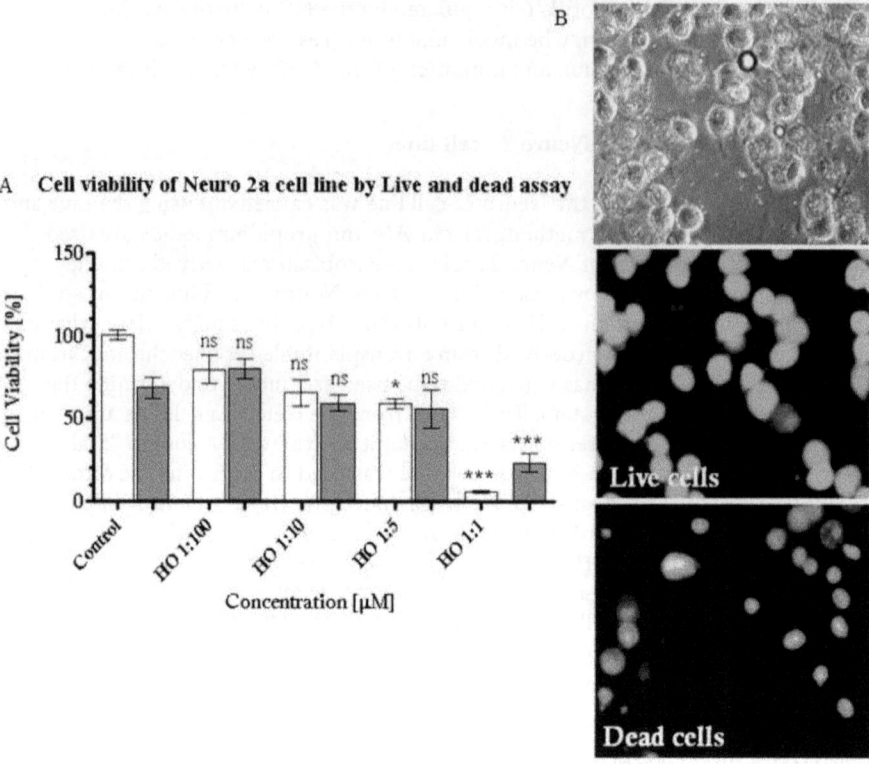

Figure 8.
A) Survival assay of HO on Neuro 2A cells for 24 h on 96-well plate. White bars, the HO was tested in the absence H_2O_2 and gray bars the HO was tested in the presence H_2O_2. The control containing water was normalized to 100% viability, significances are expressed to the control. Data presented as viability % ± SD. Significances: ns p≥0.05, *p< 0.05, **p < 0.01 and ***p < 0.001. B) Survival assay of Neuro 2A cells upon treatment with HO. Neuronal cells were plated at a density of 10,000 cells/well in 96-well tissue culture plate. After 24 h, the culture medium containing the HO was replaced with 0.2 ml of dye solution (calcein-AM and PI) and cells were observed under the microscope (Magnification 40 x). Cells treated with HO 1:5.

not a pest but a helpful organism for gardening, these nematodes can be used in normal laboratories without any special security protocols. This nematode is easy to culture, and simple toxicity screens using a normal light microscope are possible [26]. *S. feltiae* is a standard model for related environmental and agricultural vermin and pests. *S. feltiae* is normally used by gardeners as a biological defense against garden pests like flies, bugs, snails, and various other organisms. In the past few years, nematodes have grown in popularity as subjects in laboratory experiments. These small organisms are cheap, easy to handle, and they do not require any specific handling. The fact that they are useful animals in the environment with very short lifespans makes them attractive experimental subjects [27].

The effect of HO on *Steinernema feltiae* (*S. feltiae*) worms was assessed based on the nematode movement test after 24 hours of incubation. In this study, dimethyl sulfoxide (DMSO) was used as a solvent. In the activity test, this solvent was used as a control. The movement generated in the movement test was compared to the control. The HO concentrations used in this method ranged from 1:100 to 1:5. Due to the low solubility in water, the HO solution was sonicated or, alternatively, centrifuged, before it was applied to the nematodes. The two different preparations showed no toxic effect on *S. feltiae* (**Figure 9**). **Figure 9** shows that *S. feltiae* showed the most activity when treated with HO at a concentration of 1:5, with a viability

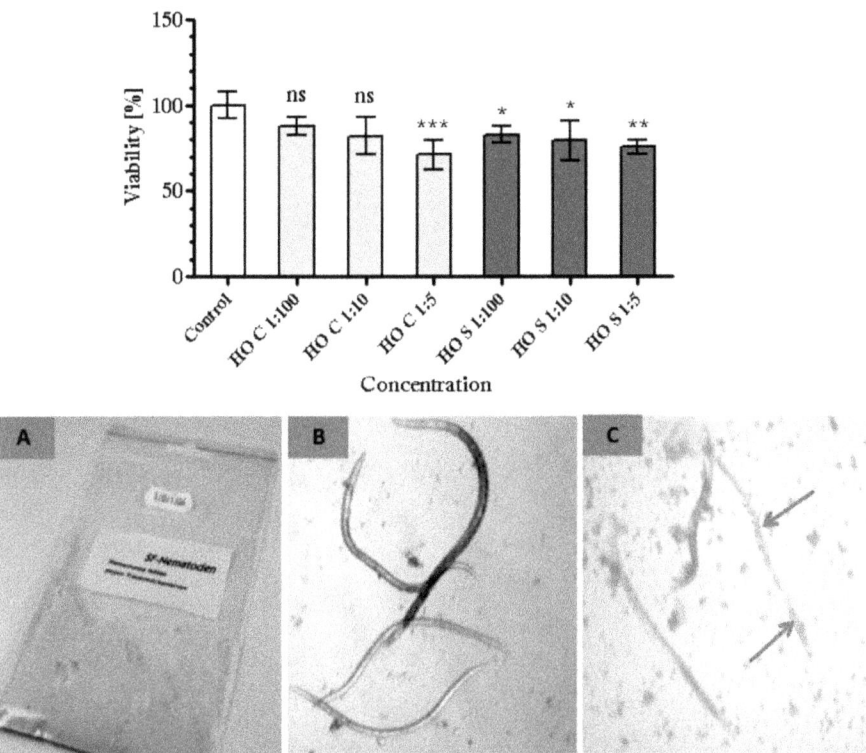

Figure 9.
Effects of HO treatment on S. feltiae after incubation for 24 hours. A) A powder cake of S. feltiae. B) Live sample of S. feltiae. C) Dead sample of S. feltiae (red arrow).

percentage of 65%. HO concentrations of 1:100 and 1:10 had no significant effect. This shows that increasing concentration of HO will increase the toxicity towards *S. feltiae*, which increases the organism's motility.

3. Conclusion

We found that HO has a strong toxic effect on the A549 cell line, with an EC_{50} value of 6.30 ppm in a CV staining assay. The Trypan Blue and CellTiter-Glo assay showed that HO also has a strong cytotoxic effect on HL-60 cells, especially at concentrations of 1:10 and 1:5. However, the results of the MTT assay showed that HO at a concentration of 1:5 had greater effectiveness than a concentration of 1:10, with a percentage of cell viability between 40 and 65%. The XTT results showed that HO at a concentration of 1:5 had a cytotoxic effect on the U937 cell line. The Hoechst staining assay showed that HO was able to increase (induce) apoptotic cells and reduce mitotic cells after 24 hours of incubation. The results also showed no detectable effect of HO on the activation and inhibition of the K562 cell line through the NF-κB pathway. Meanwhile, after HO exposure at a concentration of 1:5 and 24 hours of incubation, the Neuro 2a cell line tends to activate the apoptotic pathway. The nematicidal test showed that only at a concentration of 1:5 did HO showed significant activity, with a percentage of *S. feltiae* viability of 70%.

Acknowledgements

We would like to thank Dr. J. Lefevre for kindly providing HO for our research.

Conflict of interest

None declared.

Author details

Khairan Khairan[1,2*], Torsten Burkholz[3], Mareike Kelkel[4], Vincent Jamier[5], Karl-Herbert Schäfer[6] and Claus Jacob[7]

1 Department of Pharmacy, Universitas Syiah Kuala, Banda Aceh, Indonesia

2 Pusat Riset Obat Herbal, Universitas Syiah Kuala, Banda Aceh, Indonesia

3 Department of Applied Materials Engineering, Institute of Air Handling and Refrigeration (ILK), Dresden, Germany

4 Laboratoire de Biologie Moléculaireet Cellulaire du Cancer (LBMCC), Hôpital Kirchberg, Luxembourg

5 Leitat Technological Center, Terrassa, Spain

6 Department of Microsystems Technique, University of Applied Sciences, Zweibruecken, Germany

7 School of Pharmacy, Universitaet des Saarlandes, Saarbruecken, Germany

*Address all correspondence to: khairankhairan@unsyiah.ac.id

IntechOpen

© 2019 The Author(s). Licensee IntechOpen. This chapter is distributed under the terms of the Creative Commons Attribution License (http://creativecommons.org/licenses/by/3.0), which permits unrestricted use, distribution, and reproduction in any medium, provided the original work is properly cited. (cc) BY

References

[1] Compain P, Martin OR. Iminosugars: from synthesis to therapeutic applications. CNRS, University of Orléans, France: John Wiley & Sons; 2007. 457 p. DOI: 10.1002/9780470517437

[2] Wittop-Koning DA. History of Haarlem oil. Ceskoslovenská Farmacie. 1972;21(5):199-200

[3] Wittop-Koning DA. Contribution to the history of Haarlem oil. Pharmaceutisch Weekblad. 1972;107:165-172

[4] Lefevre JR. Du Boistesselin. Theraphy Journal. 1959;14:1044-1052

[5] Jae J, An YP, Lee SY, Kim SH, Lee MJ, Lee MS, et al. Transduced human PEP-1–heat shock protein 27 efficiently protects against brain ischemic insult. FEBS Journal. 2008;275:1296-1308. DOI: 10.1111/j.1742-4658.2008.06291.x

[6] Chan BA, Coward JIG. Chemotherapy advances in small-cell lung cancer. Journal of thoracic disease. 2013;5:565-578

[7] Stephen MR, Kehrer JP, Klotz LO. Studies on Experimental Toxicology and Pharmacology. Switzerland: Springer International Publishing; 2015. DOI: 10.1007/978-3-319-19096-9

[8] Gaugler R, Lewis E, Stuart RJ. Ecology in the service of biological control: The case of entomopathogenic nematodes. Oecologia. 1997;109:483-489. DOI: 10.1007/s004420050108

[9] Jorgensen LV, Cornett C, Justesen U, Skibsted LH, Dragsted DO. Two-electron electrochemical oxidation of quercetin and kaempferol changes only the flavonoid C-ring. Free Radical Research. 1998;29:339-350. DOI: 10.1080/10715769800300381

[10] Gaugler R. Entomopathogenic nematodes in biological control. 1st ed. Boca Raton: CRC Press; 1990. 381 p. DOI: 10.1201/9781351071741

[11] Feoktistova M, Geserick P, Leverkus M. Crystal violet assay for determining viability of cultured cells. Cold Spring Harbor Protocols. 2016;4:343-346. DOI: 10.1101/pdb.prot087379

[12] Castro-Garza J, Barrios-Garcia HB, Cruz-Vega DE, Said Fernandez S, Carranza-Rosales P, Molina-Torres CA, et al. Use of a colorimetric assay to measure differences in cytotoxicity of *Mycobacterium tuberculosis* strains. Journal of Medical Microbiology. 2007;56(6):733-737. DOI: 10.1099/jmm.0.46915-0

[13] Khairan K, Jamier V, Jacob C. Study cytotoxicity of Haarlem oil by crystal violet staining assay. Research Journal of Chemistry and Environment. 2018;22(Special Issue II):198-202. E-ISSN: 2278-4527

[14] Terry G, Riss L, Richard A, Moravec BS, Andrew LN, Sarah Duellman MS. Cell viability assay. In: Sittampalam GS, Coussens NP, Brimacombe K, editors. Assay Guidance Manual [Internet]. Eli Lilly & Company and the National Center for Advancing Translational Sciences; 2016. p. 1-31

[15] Bahi M, Jacob C, Khairan K. Cytotoxic effect of Haarlem oil on HL-60 cell line and *Steinernema feltiae*. Jurnal Kedokteran Hewan. 2016;10(2):109-114. P-ISSN : 1978-225X; E-ISSN : 2502-5600

[16] Shapiro HM. Practical Flow Cytometry. 2nd ed. New York: John Wiley & Sons; 1988. p. 129

[17] Berridge MV, Herst PM, Tan AS. Tetrazolium dyes as tools in cell biology: New insights into their cellular reduction. Biotechnology Annual Review. 2005;11:127-152. DOI: 10.1016/S1387-2656(05)11004-7

[18] Gallagher R, Collins S, Trujillo J. Characterization of the continuous, differentiating myeloid cell line (HL-60) from a patient with acute promyelocytic leukemia. Blood. 1979; 54(3):713-733

[19] Mosmann T. Rapid colorimetric assay for cellular growth and survival: Application to proliferation and cytotoxicity assays. Journal of Immunological Methods. 1983; 65(1–2):55-63

[20] Roehm NW. An improved colorimetric assay for cell proliferation and viability utilizing the tetrazolium salt XTT. Journal of Immunological Methods. 1991;142:257

[21] Susan E. Apoptosis: A review of programmed cell death. Toxicologic Pathology. 2007;35(4):495-516

[22] Santoro MG, Crisari A, Benedetto A, Amici C. Modulation of the growth of a human Erythroleukemic cell line (K562) by prostaglandins: Antiproliferative action of prostaglandin A1. Cancer Research. 1986;46:6073-6077

[23] Pobezinskaya YL, Liu Z. The role of TRADD in death receptor signaling. Cell Cycle. 2012;11(5):871-876. DOI: 10.4161/cc.11.5.19300

[24] Kaneshiro ES, Wyder MA, Wu YP, Cushion MT. Reliability of calcein acetoxy methyl-ester and ethidium homodimer or propidium iodide for viability assessment of microbes. Journal of Microbiological Methods. 1993;17:1-16. DOI: 10.1016/S0167-7012 (93)80010-4

[25] Calderon FH, Bonnefont A, Munoz FJ, Fernandez V, Videla LA, Inestrosa NC. PC12 and neuro 2a cells have different susceptibilities to acetylcholinesterase-amyloid complexes, amyloid 25-35 fragment, glutamate, and hydrogen peroxide. Journal of Neuroscience Research. 1999; 56:620-631. DOI: 10.1002/(SICI) 1097-4547(19990615)56:6<620::AID-JNR8>3.0.CO;2-F

[26] Clennan EL, Liao C. The hydroperoxysulfoniumylide. An aberration or a ubiquitous intermediate? Tetrahedron. 2006;62:10724-10728. DOI: 10.1016/j.tet.2006.07.111

[27] Buecher EJ, Popiel I. Liquid culture of the Entomogenous nematode *Steinernemafeltiae* with its bacterial Symbiont. Journal of Nematology. 1989; 21:500-504

Chapter 3

Cytotoxic Activity of Essential Oils of Some Species from Lamiaceae Family

Cuauhtémoc Pérez-González, Julia Pérez-Ramos,
Carlos Alberto Méndez-Cuesta, Roberto Serrano-Vega,
Miguel Martell-Mendoza and Salud Pérez-Gutiérrez

Abstract

Cancer is considered one of the most lethal diseases in the world, with a prevalence of 439.2 cases and 163.5 deaths per 100,000 inhabitants, in the period from 2011 to 2015; this disease has a greater impact in underdeveloped countries. For the treatment of this disease, a combination of chemotherapy with surgery or radiation is generally used, however, it is not exempt from adverse effects or resistance of the tumor to this type of treatment, for this reason the search for new treatments is constant. The plants are a possible source to achieve this; Lamiaceae is a family of plants widely distributed on the planet and has been used traditionally for the treatment of different diseases, and various essential oils with the potential for cancer treatment have been isolated from this species. The scope of this review is to present 46 essential oils isolated from different species of Lamiaceae which have been tested against different cancer cell lines.

Keywords: essential oils, Lamiaceae family, cytotoxic activity

1. Introduction

Cancer is a complex disease due to its multiple etiologies, and cancer cells are different to normal cells in many ways. The main characteristics of cancer cells are the cell growth out-of-control in a part of the body that spreads to surrounding tissue, and cancer cells are less specialized than the normal cells. Cancer cells ignore signals that normally tell cells to stop dividing or that begin the process of apoptosis. Also, these cells frequently evade the immune system.

These cells influence the normal cells, molecules, and blood vessels which feed tumors supplying with oxygen and nutrients, which they need to grow. These blood vessels also remove waste products from tumors [1].

Cancer has a large global impact; between 2011 and 2015, the number of new cases of cancer was 439.2 per 100,000 habitants, the cancer mortality rate was 163.5 per 100,000, and cancer mortality was higher for men than women [2].

In 2012, approximately 57% of new cancer cases were detected in less developed countries such as those in Central America and some parts of Africa and Asia, where 65% of cancer deaths occurred. In 2030, it is expected that the number of new cancer cases will rise to 23.6 million [2].

In 2017, it was estimated that in the USA, national expenditures for cancer care were $147.3 billion dollars, and the cost will rise with the increase in cancer prevalence and population age.

Currently, many types of cancer treatment are used. Most patients with cancer undergo a combination of treatments, such as surgery with chemotherapy, radiation, immunotherapy, targeted therapy, or hormone therapy. Chemotherapy is one of the most common cancer treatments, but the drugs used produce severe side effects, such as nausea, vomiting, and alopecia, among others, which diminish the quality of life of the patients.

The use of plants in the treatment of many diseases is an ancient practice that has an increased use in recent years. Medicinal plants are a source of compounds with biological activities as anticancer agents, and over 50% of the drugs used in the clinical treatment of cancer, such as Taxol, camptothecin, vincristine, and vinblastine, were obtained from natural sources.

Essential oils (EOs) are a highly complex, volatile, and odorous mixture. The main components are monoterpenes, sesquiterpenes, and aromatic compounds. EOs are obtained mainly by steam distillation [3]. EOs have several activities, such as antimicrobial, anti-inflammatory, bactericidal, antiviral, fungicidal, antiangiogenic, and antitumor activities [4].

The Lamiaceae family comprises 240 genera and 7200 species distributed around the world. Most members of this family are perennial or annual herbs with square stems and are woody shrubs or subshrubs. This family is characterized by aromatic plants, which are widely used as culinary herbs, such as basil, mint, oregano, and sage. Species of this family are important ornamental and medicinal plants and are considered one of the most important sources of EOs of economic importance. In fact, different studies suggest that several EOs obtained from this family have demonstrated cytotoxic activity against different cell cancer lines and could be used as a preventive and alternative treatment for cancer [5]. Several EOs obtained from plants of this family contain high amounts of monoterpenes, such as thymol, carvacrol, 1,8-cineole, and limonene, among others, and the cytotoxic activity of some of these compounds has been studied.

The aim of this review is to provide a critical overview of the research on the traditional medicine basis, cytotoxic properties, cancer cell lines targeted, and composition of EOs isolated from plants belonging to the Lamiaceae family.

2. Satureja

Satureja L., which includes approximately 38 species in the Mediterranean region, is used in folk medicine to treat various ailments, such as cramps, muscle pains, nausea, indigestion, diarrhea, and infectious diseases, as well as for its antioxidant, cytotoxic, antidiabetes, anti-HIV, antihyperlipidemic, reproduction-stimulating, expectorant, and vasodilatory effects.

S. cilicica P.H. Davis is an endemic species of Turkey. EO from aerial parts of *S. cilicica* collected in Turkey was obtained in a yield of 0.69% v/w. The main identified compounds were *p*-cymene (17.68%), carvacrol (14.02%), γ-terpinene (11.23%), and thymol (8.76%). The cytotoxic activity of the EO was determined in the MCF-7 (breast cancer) cell line, revealing an IC_{50} value of 268 μg/mL [6].

S. sahandica Bornm. aerial parts were collected in Iran. The EO yield was 0.52% (w/w). Thymol (40%), γ-terpinene (28%), and ρ-cymene (22%) were the main compounds. The cytotoxicity of the EO in MCF-7, Vero, SW480 (adenocarcinoma cell), and JET 3 (choriocarcinoma cells) cell lines was dose-dependent, with IC_{50} values of 15.6, 15.6, 125, and 250 μg/mL, respectively [7].

S. intermedia L. is used to treat diarrhea, nausea, cramps, muscle pain, indigestion, and infectious diseases. A sample was collected in Iran, and the major components were thymol (34.5%), γ-terpinene (18.2%), and *p*-cymene (10.5%). The cytotoxic activity was tested in the 5637 (urinary bladder carcinoma) and KYSE (human Asian squamous cell carcinoma) cell lines, and an IC_{50} value of 156 μg/mL was obtained in both cases [8].

S. intermedia C.A. Mey EO was obtained from the aerial parts collected in Fars Province, Iran. The main components of the EO were γ-terpinene (37.1%), thymol (30.2%), p-cymene (16.2%), limonene (3.9%), α-terpinene (3.3%), and myrcene (2.5%). The EO showed an $IC_{50} \geq 50$ μg/mL in the Hep-G2 (hepatocellular carcinoma) and MCF-7 cell lines. The effect was evaluated by the crystal violet staining method [9].

S. khuzistanica Jamzad is used as analgesic and antiseptic in Iran. The aerial parts were collected in southern Iran. The EO was analyzed by GC/FID and GC/MS. The EO yield was 0.42% (w/w), and the main component was carvacrol (92.87%). MTT cytotoxicity assay was employed. The EO reduced the viability of Vero, SW480 (colon adenocarcinoma), MCF-7, and JET 3 cell lines, with IC_{50} values of 31.2, 62.5, 125, and 125 μg/mL, respectively [10].

S. montana subsp. *pisidica* L. is used for its antiseptic, aromatic, carminative, digestive, and expectorant properties and in the treatment of insect bites. The major compounds of the EOs obtained from the aerial parts collected in Korab and Galicica were carvacrol, thymol, carvacrol methyl ether, and β-linalool. The cytotoxic effect of the EOs was tested against MDA-MB-361, MDA-MB-453 (human mammary metastatic carcinoma), HeLa, LS174 (human colorectal adenocarcinoma), and MRC5 (fibroblast of lung cells) cell lines. The EO from Korab had higher activity than the oil from Galicica, particularly against the HeLa and MDA-MB-453 cell lines, with IC_{50} values of 63.5 and 72.3 μg/mL, respectively [11].

S. bakhtiarica Bunge. is traditionally used for its antiseptic, carminative, stimulant, diaphoretic, diuretic, anesthetic, antispasmodic, analgesic, antioxidant, sedative, and antimicrobial properties. *S. bakhtiarica* is an endemic plant in the southern region of Iran. Leaves of *S. bakhtiarica* were collected in the Fars Province of Iran. The chemical composition of the EO was determined by GC/MS, and the main components were phenol (56.35%), thymol (13.82%), p-cymene (8.79%), and carvacrol (2.88%). An MTT cytotoxicity assay was used to test the effect of the EO on HEK (human normal embryonic kidney cells), MDA-MB-231, and SKOV3 (human ovary cancer cells) cell lines. The EO showed antitumor activity against the SKOV3 and MDA-MB-231 cell lines (IC_{50} values of 74.6 μg/mL and IC_{50} of 83.7 μg/mL, respectively) [12].

3. Nepeta

N. schiraziana Boiss possesses medicinal properties such as antitussive, diaphoretic, antispasmodic, antiasthmatic, diuretic, emmenagogue, and antipyretic effects. The aerial parts of *N. schiraziana* were collected in Iran. The compounds identified in the EO were 1,8-cineole (33.67%), germacrene D (11.45%), β-caryophyllene (9.88%), caryophyllene oxide (7.34%), α-pinene (4.59%), and camphor (3.75%). The EO was tested against Hep-G2 (IC_{50} of 85.74 μg/mL) and MCF-7 (IC_{50} of 32.56 μg/mL) cell lines [13].

N. rtanjensis Diklić & Milojević is found only in a few localities of Mt. Rtanj in northeast Serbia. This plant has antibacterial, antifungal, allelopathic, and phytotoxic activities. *N. rtanjensis* was cultivated at the University of Belgrade, Serbia. Chemical analysis revealed that *N. rtanjensis* EO contains *trans,cis*-nepetalactone (71.66%), *cis,trans*-nepetalactone (17.21%), α-pinene (3.28%), 2-methoxy-paracresol (1.85%), and α-copaene (0.86%). Cytotoxic assays were performed on five tumor cell lines (HeLa, A549, lung adenocarcinoma cells; LS-174, human colon cancer cells; K562, human myelogenous leukemia cells; and MDA-MB-231), and the IC_{50} values were 0.050, 0.064, 0.097, 0.052, and 0.097 μL/mL, respectively [14].

N. sintenisii Bornm. The EO is used in Iranian folk medicine as a diuretic, antitussive, and antispasmodic treatment. The plant was collected in Neyshabur, Khorasan-Razavi, Iran. The yield of EO was 0.5% v/w, and the composition was determined by using GC/MS. The major compounds were 4aα,7α,7aβ-nepetalactone (51.74%), β-farnesene (12.26), 4aα,7α,7aα-nepetalactone (8.01%), germacrene D (5.01%), and 4α,7α,7aα-nepetalactone (3.71%). The cytotoxicity was evaluated against four cell lines, A2780, HeLa, LS180, and MCF-7. The IC_{50} values were 51.98, 20.37, 42.64, and 43.75 μg/mL, respectively [15].

N. menthoides Boiss & Buhse is an herbaceous aromatic plant endemic to northwest Iran and has been used to treat gastrodynia, insomnia, high blood pressure, bone pain, and rheumatism. The aerial parts were collected in Ardabil, Iran. The EO was analyzed by GC/MS. The major components were 4a-α,7β,7a-α-nepetalactone (18.39%), 4a-α,7α,7a-α-nepetalactone (17.57%), 1,8-cineol (16.66%), and geranyl acetate (7.0%). The cytotoxic activity was evaluated against HT-29 (colon carcinoma), Caco-2 (colorectal adenocarcinoma), T47D (breast ductal carcinoma), and NIH-3 T3 cell lines using the MTT method. The IC_{50} values were 30.7, 19.37, and 32.24 μg/mL, respectively [16].

4. Thymus

The genus *Thymus* consists of approximately 215 species distributed throughout Europe, Asia, and North Africa. Most of these plants are important in food, pharmaceutical, and cosmetic fields. Many species have been investigated for their preservative effects on foods, protecting the food from lipid peroxidation. In traditional medicine, the leaves and flowering aerial parts of *Thymus* species have been used extensively for their tonic, antiseptic, antitussive, and carminative properties in the treatment of colds, coughs, sore throats, cystitis, insomnia, bronchitis, and indigestion.

T. munbyanus Boiss. & Reut. is an endemic species of North Africa and is used as an antimicrobial, antioxidant, and antiproliferative agent. Fresh aerial parts of *T. munbyanus* were collected in Hennaya, Algeria. The EO was analyzed by GC and GC/MS. The main components of the oil were carvacrol (71%), *p*-cymene (8.3%), and ϒ-terpinene (5.9%). The *T. munbyanus* EO showed antiproliferative activity against the human acute monocytic leukemia cell line (THP-1, 100 μg/mL) using MTT assay [17].

T. munbyanus subsp. *coloratus* Boiss. and Reut. has been reported to be effective against cough, colds, influenza, sore throat, abdominal bloating, and endocrine gland diseases and as a depurative agent. Inflorescences and vegetative parts (stems + leaves) of *T. munbyanus* subsp. *coloratus* collected in Algeria yielded 0.2% and 0.1% w/w EO, respectively. The principal components of the EO from flowers were borneol (44.8%), camphor (5.7%), 1,8-cineole (6.0%), and germacrene D (5.0%). The major constituents of the EO from aerial parts were borneol (31.2%), camphor (13.6%), and camphene (7.5%). The cytotoxic activity was tested, and the EO from flowers showed higher activity against the A375 (IC_{50} of 46.95 μg/mL), T98G (human glioblastoma multiforme; IC_{50} of 51.54 μg/mL), and MDA-MB-231 (IC_{50} of 97.27 μg/mL) cell lines than that from leaves and stems. The EO from leaves and stems was cytotoxic against T98G (IC_{50} of 91.83 µg/mL), MDA-MB-231 (IC_{50} of 84.77 µg/mL), and A375 (IC_{50} > 100 µg/mL) cell lines [18].

T. carmanicus Jalas is used in Iranian folk medicine in the treatment of rheumatism and skin disorders and as an antibacterial agent. Aerial parts were collected from Iran, and the EO was obtained in 2.67% w/w yield. The main components were carvacrol (51.0%), thymol (20.84%), borneol (6.80%), cymene (6.25%), γ-terpinene (5.50%), and β-myrcene (1.63%). The IC_{50} value was 0.44 µL/mL in KB cell line (oral carcinoma) [19].

T. vulgaris L. is reported to have antiseptic, antispasmodic, antimicrobial, antioxidant, anti-inflammatory, and anticancer effects. This plant was cultivated in Helwan University Cairo/Egypt. EO was obtained from the fresh and aerial parts with a yield of 0.21% v/w. The major constituents were p-cymene (31.62% v/w), γ-terpenine (17.72% v/w), thymyl methyl ether (9.83% v/w), and thymol (7.38% v/w). The cytotoxic effect of EO was tested in four cell lines: A-549, IC_{50} of 7.22 µg/mL; HCT-116, IC_{50} of 3.61 µg/mL; CaCo-2, IC_{50} of 1.93 µg/mL; and MCF-7, IC_{50} of 9.52 µg/mL [20].

5. Mentha

The genus *Mentha* includes 20 species found all over the world. Most *Mentha* species are perennial, contain essential oils, and are widely cultivated as industrial crops for essential oil production. Many EO chemotypes have a distinct aromatic flavor conferred by different terpene. The whole herb of these species has been used to extract many compounds that have been evaluated as antifungal, antiviral, antimicrobial, insecticidal, antioxidant, antiamoebic, antihemolytic, antiallergenic, and antitumoral agents.

M. spicata L. is a medicinal plant, and its EO inhibits free radical reactions, retards the oxidative rancidity of lipids, and shows antimicrobial and antitumor activities. The major compounds in the EO from *M. spicata* collected in China were carvone (65.33%), limonene (18.19%), dihydrocarvone (2.97%), and camphene (2.34%). The cytotoxicity was evaluated in a HeLa cell line, and an IC_{50} value of approximately 2.08 µg/mL was obtained [21].

M. piperita L. is commonly known as peppermint. It is widely grown in temperate areas of the world, particularly Europe, North America, and North Africa. The EO extracted from its aerial parts was analyzed by GC/MS, and the main component was menthol (47.5%). The cytotoxic activity of the EO was tested against HeLa, A549, and MRC-5 (human fibroblast lung cells) using MTT assay. The IC_{50} values were 165.24, 183.00, and 197.08 µg/mL, respectively. EO was obtained from *M. piperita* collected in Guatemala in a yield of 0.50% w/w. The IC_{50} values of the EO against the AGS, A375, and A431 cell lines were 0.35, 0.40, and 0.23 µL/mL, respectively [22].

M. pulegium L. is commonly known as pennyroyal. This plant is traditionally used in the treatment of infectious diseases. Analysis of the EO by GC/MS revealed pulegone (68.7%) as the main component. The cytotoxic activity of the EO was tested against HeLa, A549, and MRC-5 cell lines using MTT assay. The IC_{50} values of the EO were 168.58, 253.64, and 189.48 µg/mL, respectively [23].

6. Ocimum

The genus *Ocimum* includes approximately 150 species, comprising annual and perennial herbs and shrubs native to the tropical and subtropical regions of Asia, Africa, and Central and South America. *Ocimum* species are commercially cultivated aromatic crops in India and other countries for the EO and high-value aromatic chemicals used extensively in food, perfumery, cosmetic and pharmaceutical preparations, and as spices. *Ocimum* species are known for their diverse use in folk medicine for the treatment of various gastric and urinary diseases, insomnia, inflammation, and constipation due to their diverse biological actions, such as carminative, stimulant, antiseptic, antimicrobial, antioxidant, antipyretic, insecticidal, and antispasmodic activities.

Ocimum basilicum L. grows in several regions all over the world and is traditionally used to treat anxiousness, grippe, infectious diseases, headaches, coughs, acne, diarrhea, constipation, warts, worms, and kidney malfunction. EO from its leaves has insecticidal, pesticidal, antibacterial, antioxidant, antiviral, antifungal, antiulcer, cytotoxic, and larvicidal activities.

Plants were collected in Guatemala, and the yield of EO was 0.33% w/w. The main components of the EO were methyl cinnamate (70.1%), linalool (17.5%), β-elemene (2.6%), and camphor (1.52%). The IC_{50} values of the EO against AGS (epithelial gastric adenocarcinoma), A375 (epithelial malignant melanoma), and A431 (epithelial squamous carcinoma) cell lines were 0.39, 0.36, and 0.34 μL/mL, respectively [22].

This oil was also tested against HeLa (cervical adenocarcinoma cells; IC_{50} of 90.5 μg/mL) and HEp-2 (human epithelioma; IC_{50} of 96.3 μg/mL) cell lines [24]. In *O basilicum* L. collected in Egypt (yield of 0.85% v/w), the major components were estragole (75.45%), 1,8-cineole (7.56%), linalool (5.01%), trans-anethole (3.72%), and methyleugenol (3.48%). The anticancer activity was assessed in HL-60 (promyelocytic leukemia) and NB4 (acute promyelocytic leukemia) cell lines. The EO was tested at doses of 200 μg/mL in both cell lines and killed 82.33% of HL-60 cells and 73.38% of NB4 cells [25].

O. canum Sims. is used in traditional Indian medicinal for treating diabetes, cold, fever, inflammation, and headaches. The EO was obtained from its leaves. The main components were camphor (39.77%), naphtalene (7.37%), valencene (5.80%), α-pinene (5.59%), camphene (5.20%), and caryophyllene (5.62%). The cytotoxic activity of the EO was tested against MCF-7 cells (IC_{50} of 60 μg/mL) [26].

O. kilimandscharicum Guerke, popularly known as "Basil African blue," is a semi-evergreen shrub native to East Africa and used in traditional medicine for the treatment of constipation, abdominal pain, cough, and diarrhea. The chemical composition of the EO was determined by GC/MS, and the main components were camphor (51.81%), 1,8-cineole (20.13%), and limonene (11.23%). The EO was evaluated against OVCAR-03 cell line (human epithelial ovarian adenocarcinoma) using a sulforhodamine B (SRB) colorimetric assay, with an IC_{50} of 31.90 μg/mL [27].

7. Salvia

The Salvia genus comprises more than 960 species, which are known as Sage in folk medicine and have been used in the treatment of different ailments, such as stomach pain, diarrhea, fever, inflammation, headaches, bruises, and sprains.

Aerial parts of these plants usually contain flavonoids, triterpenoids, and essential oils. Diterpenoids are the main compounds in the roots. These compounds show a variety of activities, and different pharmacological models have been used to explain their mechanisms of activity.

S. officinalis L. is used in traditional medicine to treat microbial infections, cancer, malaria, and inflammation and to disinfect homes after sickness. This plant was collected in south-central Italy in 2008–2009. The leaves were used to obtain an EO, the composition of which was determined by GC/MS, with a yield of 0.55–2.2% on a dry mass basis. The main components were α-thujone, camphor, borneol, γ-muurolene, and sclareol. The anticancer activity was tested in the cell lines M14, A375, and A2058. The IC_{50} values were 8.2, 12.1, and 11.7 μg/mL, respectively [28].

S. macrosiphon Boiss is used for treating infection; rheumatoid arthritis; chronic pain; inflammatory, cardiovascular, and cerebrovascular diseases; and as an antioxidant, acetylcholinesterase-inhibiting, antinociceptive, anti-inflammatory, antidepressant, anxiolytic, antitumor, and cytotoxic agent. S. macrosiphon was collected in Iran. The aerial parts yielded 0.2% v/w of EO. Analysis of the EO showed that linalool (19%), β-cedrene (14.64%), and β-elemene (13.33%) were the major components. The effect of the EO on the proliferation of cell lines MCF-7, MDA-MB-231, and T47D was assessed, and the IC_{50} values were 0.155, 0.145, and 0.093 μg/mL, respectively [29].

S. lavandulifolia Vahl is a medicinal plant native to the Iberian Peninsula. It is used to treat gastric problems and inflammatory disorders. The composition of its EO was determined by GC/MS, and camphor (29.1%) was the main component. The cytotoxic activity of the EO was tested against HeLa, A549, and MRC-5 cell lines using MTT assay. The IC_{50} values of the EO were 133.56, 140.10, and 131.50 μg/mL, respectively [30].

8. Lavandula

The genus *Lavandula* includes more than 20 species, and the EOs from the species of this genus have been applied in food, pharmaceutical, and agricultural industries as biological products. Four medicinal plants of this genus (*L. vera* DC, *L. angustifolia* Miller, *L. latifolia* Medikus, and *L. hybrida* Rev) were collected in Italy. The EO constituents were analyzed, and the major compounds were as follows: linalool (36.15%), linalyl acetate (17.08%), and terpinen-4-ol (16.13%) in *L. vera* DC; linalool (56.57%) and camphor (10.01%) in *L. angustifolia* Miller; linalool (34.43%), linalyl acetate (24.36%), and camphor (8.84%) in *L. latifolia* Medikus; and linalool (39.24%), linalyl acetate (22.88%), and 1,8-cineole (6.74%) in *L. hybrida* Rev. The EOs were tested in Caco-2 cell line (epithelial colorectal adenocarcinoma), and the cytotoxic effect of EOs was very low [31].

L. angustifolia Mill. was collected in the southeastern region of Brazil. The yield obtained for its EO was 0.28% (w/w), and the major components were borneol (22.4%), epi-α-muurolol (13.4%), α-bisabolol (13.1%), precocene I (13%), and eucalyptol (7.9%). The cytotoxic activity was tested in the cell line GM07492-A and was observed only at a high concentration (IC_{50} of 243.7 μg/mL) [32].

L. angustifolia Mill was collected in Bulgaria. Analysis of the EO extracted from its aerial parts revealed linalool (40.3%) as the main component. The cytotoxic activity of the EO was tested against HeLa (IC_{50} of 80.62 μg/mL), A549 (88.90 of μg/mL), and MRC-5 (75.19 of μg/mL) cell lines using MTT assay [30].

9. Origanum

Origanum species are herbaceous perennial shrubs native to Europe and North Africa. These plants have aromatic leaves. This genus includes important culinary plants, such as marjoram and oregano.

O. onites Elmalı is used in Turkey as a condiment or aromatic tea, and a sample of this species was collected in Antalya, Turkey. EO was obtained from the herbal parts of the plant. The composition was determined by GC/MS; the main components were carvacrol (24.52%), thymol (15.66%), and linalool (50.53%).

The cytotoxicity of the EO, thymol, and carvacrol was determined against hepatoma G2 cells (Hep G2), and the IC_{50} values were 149.12, 53.09, and 60.1 µg/mL, respectively [33].

O. vulgare L. is used in traditional medicine for treating colds, indigestion, and upset stomach. The plant was collected in Guatemala, and the yield of EO was 0.66% w/w. The IC_{50} values of the EO against epithelial gastric adenocarcinoma, epithelial malignant melanoma, and epithelial squamous carcinoma were 0.18, 0.09, and 0.08 µL/mL, respectively [22].

O. vulgare L. is commonly known as oregano and *O. majorana* L. as sweet marjoram. The EOs from both species have antioxidant and antimicrobial properties; these plants were collected in Faisalabad, Pakistan, in July–August 2008. The EOs were analyzed by GC and GC/MS. The main components of the EO from *O. vulgare* were terpinen-4-ol (20.9%), linalool (15.7%), linalyl acetate (13.9%), limonene (13.4%), and α-terpineol (8.57%). The major compounds in the EO from *O. majorana* were thymol (21.6%), carvacrol (18.8%), and α-terpineol (8.57%).

The cytotoxic activity of the EO from *O. vulgare* was tested against MCF-7, prostate cancer (LNCaP), and NIH3T3 cell lines. The IC_{50} values were 70, 85.3, and 300.5 µg/mL, respectively. The IC_{50} values for the EO from *O. majorana* were 100, 90.1, and 320.3 µg/mL, respectively [34].

The EO obtained from *O. vulgare* collected in Córdoba, Argentina, was analyzed by GC/MS. Analysis of the chemical composition showed carvacrol and thymol as the predominant compounds. The cytotoxicity activity was evaluated in cultured A549 cells, and this oil reduced the viability of the cells (IC_{50} of 2.25 µg/mL) [35].

Tetradenia riparia Hochst Codd is used in traditional medicinal to treat cough, dropsy, diarrhea, fever, headaches, malaria, and toothaches. The main components of its EO were *E,E*-farnesol (15%), aromadendrene oxide (14.7%), and dronabinol (11%). The cytotoxic activity was tested against HT29 (IC_{50} of 6.93 µg/mL), MCF-7 (IC_{50} of 129.57 µg/mL), HeLa (IC_{50} of 155 µg/mL), HepG-2 (IC_{50} of 149.97 µg/mL), glioblastoma (M059; IC_{50} of 217.97 µg/mL), U343 (IC_{50} of 221.30 µg/mL), and U251 (IC_{50} of 109.90 µg/mL) cells using an XTT-based toxicology assay kit [36].

T. riparia leaves were collected in Umuarama, Brazil. 9β,13β-Epoxy-7-abietene (1) was isolated from the EO. The cytotoxic activities of the EO and (1) were determined by MTT assay in the MDA-MB-435, HCT-8, SF-295, and HL-60 cell lines. The EO and compound (1), at concentrations of 50 µg/mL and 25 µg/mL, respectively, showed high cytotoxic potential against the cell lines SF-295 (78.06% and 94.80%), HCT-8 (85.00% and 86.54%), and MDA-MB-435 (59.48% and 45.43%) [37].

Ajuga chamaepitys L. Schreb grows in the Mediterranean region and is used as a diuretic and emmenagogue. This plant was collected in Rocca Mattei, Italy, and the composition of the EO isolated from the aerial parts was determined by GC and GC/MS. Ethyl linoleate (13.7%), germacrene D (13.4%), kaurene (8.4%), β-pinene (6.8%), and phytol (5.3%) were the major components. The EO had moderate cytotoxic activity against the MDA-MB-231 cell line (IC_{50} of 36.88 µg/mL) and an IC_{50} value of 60.48 µg/mL against the human colon carcinoma cell line (HCT116) [38].

Ziziphora tenuior L. is used in Jordan for the treatment of stomachache, dysentery, and fever. The EO was obtained in 0.72% yield, and the composition was determined using GC/MS; pulegone (46.8%) and *p*-menth-3-en-8-ol (12.5%) were the major compounds. The EO was tested against HepG2 cell line, and cytotoxicity was determined using MTT assay. The IC_{50} value obtained for the EO was 1.25 µL/mL [39].

Sideritis montana L. subsp. *montana* is used as a diuretic and digestive aid. *S. montana* was collected in Camerino, Italy. The EO (yield of 0.07%) was analyzed using GC/MS, and the major compounds were germacrene D (20.8%), bicyclogermacrene (13.3%), and 8,13-abietadien-18-ol (10.2%). The cytotoxicity was tested against MDA-MB-231 and HCT116 cell lines with IC$_{50}$ values of 32.32 and 31.84 μg/mL, respectively [40].

Stachys annua L. is a perennial herb and small shrub. In the folk medicine of central Italy, its aerial parts have been used as anticatarrhal, antipyretic, tonic, and vulnerary (wound healing) agents. The EO isolated from its aerial parts was analyzed by GC/MS, and the major components were phytol (9.8%), germacrene D (9.2%), spathulenol (8.5%), and bicyclogermacrene (5.8%). The cytotoxic activity of the EO was determined by MTT assay. Analysis of the cytotoxicity against the HCT116, A375, and MDA-MB-231 cell lines showed IC$_{50}$ values of 23.5, 37.2, and 41.5 μg/mL, respectively [41].

Plectranthus amboinicus Lour Spreng is cultivated in home gardens and is used in India for the treatment of cough, chronic asthma, and hiccough. The leaves of *P. amboinicus* were collected from a medicinal plant garden in Tamil, India. The cytotoxic activity of the EO was tested using MTT assay against the MCF-7 and HT-29 cell lines, and the IC$_{50}$ values were 53 and 87 μg/mL, respectively [42].

Zhumeria majdae Rech. F. & Wendelbo is a medicinal plant endemic to Iran that is under the threat of extinction. This plant has been used as a curative agent for stomachache, flatulence, diarrhea, indigestion, cold, and headache, for wound healing and treatment of painful menstruation, and as an antiseptic. The aerial parts of *Z. majdae* were collected at five locations in Iran (S1, S2, S3, S4, and S5). The major components were trans-linalool oxide (18.7%), linalool (29.6%), and camphor (27.4%) at S1; trans-linalool oxide (28.6%), linalool (24.4%), and camphor (27.2%) at S2; trans-linalool oxide (16.2%), linalool (34.2%), and camphor (27.7%) at S3; trans-linalool oxide (14.6%), linalool (33.9%), and camphor (26.1%) at S4; and trans-linalool oxide (7.6%), linalool (34.6%), and camphor (34.7%) at S5. The cytotoxicity of the EOs was measured using MTT assay against A375 and MCF7 cell lines, with IC$_{50}$ values of 746 (S1), 666 (S2), 624 (S3), 779 (S4), and 718 (S5) μg/mL and 674 (S1), 717 (S2), 732 (S3), 646 (S4), and 642 (S5), μg/mL, respectively [43].

Cedronella canariensis L. Webb & Berthel. (syn. *Dracocephalum canariense* L.) is present in the Canary Islands. It is a perennial herb, sometimes shrubby. The plant is used in traditional medicine as an anticatarrhal, tonic, antimicrobial, analgesic, carminative, diuretic, hypoglycemiant, hypotensive, and anti-inflammatory agent and decongestant of the respiratory tract. The EO was obtained from the aerial parts of *C. canariensis* collected in El Monte de las Mercedes, Canary Islands, Spain, in 2013 (yield of 2.5%). The EO was analyzed by GC/FID and GC/MS; pinocarvone (58.0%) and α-pinene (10.8%) were the main constituents. The cytotoxicity of the EO was evaluated against A345 (IC$_{50}$ of 4.3 μg/mL), MDA-MB-231 (IC$_{50}$ of 7.3 μg/mL), and HCT 116 (IC$_{50}$ of 11.4 μg/mL) cell lines by MTT assay [44].

Rosmarinus officinalis L. EO is used as an antibacterial, cytotoxic, antimutagenic, antioxidant, antiphlogistic, and chemopreventive agent. The EO (yield of 0.23% w/w) was extracted from the plant collected in Guatemala. The IC$_{50}$ values of the EO against AGS, A375, and A431 cell lines were 0.21, 0.24, and 0.41 μL/mL, respectively [22].

Teucrium yemense Delfi. possesses antifungal, antibacterial, larvicidal, antispasmodic, antioxidant, anti-inflammatory, antiulcer, hypoglycemic, antiacetylcholinesterase, and hepatoprotective activities. Its leaves were collected in two different provinces of Yemen: Dhamar (TY-d) and Taiz (TY-t). The EOs were analyzed, and the most abundant constituents of TY-d were (*E*)-caryophyllene (11.2%), α-humulene (4.0%), γ-selinene (5.5%), 7-epi-α-selinene (20.1%), and caryophyllene oxide (20.1%). The major compounds in TY-t were α-pinene (6.6%), (*E*)-caryophyllene (19.1%), α-humulene (6.4%), δ-cadinene (6.5%), caryophyllene oxide (4.3%), α-cadinol (9.5%), and shyobunol (4.6%). TY-d was active against the HT-29 cell line with an IC$_{50}$ value of 43.7 μg/mL. TY-t was active against the MCF-7 and MDA-MB-231 cell lines (IC$_{50}$ of 24.4 and 59.9 μg/mL, respectively) [45].

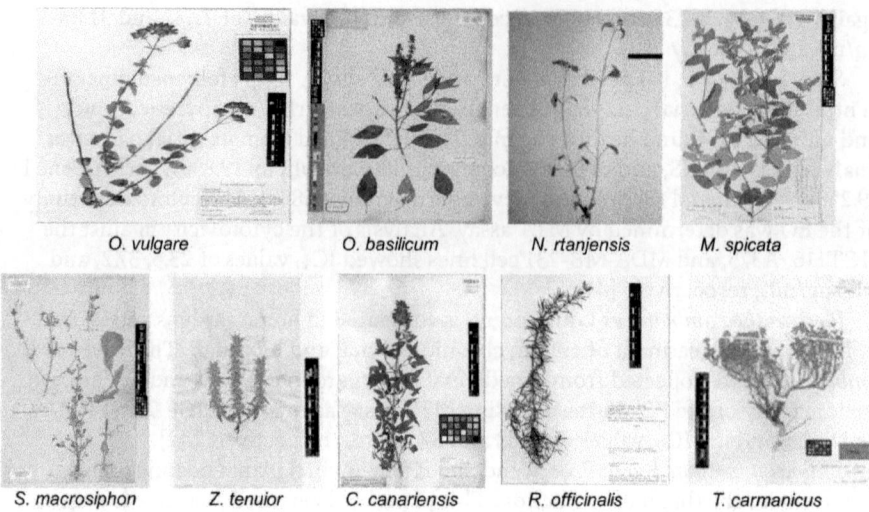

Figure 1.
Plants whose EOs present remarkable cytotoxic activity. Images taken from [48]. Image of N. rtanjensis taken from [49].

Premna microphylla Turcz. is broadly distributed in the eastern, middle, and southern regions of China. Leaves of *P. microphylla* are used to treat dysentery, appendicitis, and infections for their antioxidant and cytotoxic activities. The plant was collected in China. The EO was obtained with a yield of 0.31% w/w. The major components were blumenol C (49.7%), β-cedrene (6.1%), limonene (3.8%), α-guaiene (3.3%), cryptone (3.1%), and α-cyperone (2.7%). The EO was tested for its cytotoxic activity against HepG2 and MCF-7 cells, with IC_{50} values of 0.072 and 0.188 mg/mL, respectively [46].

Dracocephalum kotschyi Boiss is native to Iran. In traditional medicine, it is used to treat headaches, congestion, and liver disorders and for its antihyperlipidemic and anti-epimastigotic effects. The herb *D. kotschyi* is locally known as "Sama" in Lorestan Province. Aerial parts of wild *D. kotschyi* Boiss were collected in western Iran. A yellowish fragrant oil was obtained (yield of 0.16% w/w). The principal components of the EO were geranial (12.08%), α-pinene (10.34%), geraniol acetate (10.27%), geraniol (9.55%), neral (8.9%), limonene (6.95%), β-myrcene (3.42%), and β-pinene (2.18%). The IC_{50} against HeLa cell line was 26.4 μg/mL [47].

The National Cancer Institute of the USA (NCI) has screened approximately 100,000 compounds and 50,000 natural product extracts for potential anticancer agents [47]. The NCI considers a compound or an extract to have potential anticancer activity if it has an IC_{50} value of 4 or 30 μg/mL, respectively. Therefore, according to the NCI, the EOs described in this review with remarkable cytotoxic activity are those obtained from *O. basilicum*, *S. sahandica*, *O. vulgare*, *N. rtanjensis*, *M. spicata*, *S. macrosiphon*, *Z. tenuior*, *C. canariensis*, *R. officinalis*, and *T. carmanicus* (**Figure 1**).

Author details

Cuauhtémoc Pérez-González, Julia Pérez-Ramos, Carlos Alberto Méndez-Cuesta, Roberto Serrano-Vega, Miguel Martell-Mendoza and Salud Pérez-Gutiérrez*
Universidad Autónoma Metropolitana-Xochimilco, Ciudad de México, Mexico

*Address all correspondence to: msperez@correo.xoc.uam.mx

IntechOpen

© 2019 The Author(s). Licensee IntechOpen. This chapter is distributed under the terms of the Creative Commons Attribution License (http://creativecommons.org/licenses/by/3.0), which permits unrestricted use, distribution, and reproduction in any medium, provided the original work is properly cited. (cc) BY

References

[1] Hanahan D, Weinberg RA. Hallmarks of cancer: The next generation. Cell. 2011;**144**:646-674. DOI: 10.1016/j.cell.2011.02.013

[2] https://www.wcrf.org/dietandcancer/cancer-trends/data-cancer-frequency-country consulted February 11, 2019

[3] Bakkali F, Averbeck S, Averbeck D, Idaomar M. Biological effects of essential oils—A review. Food and Chemical Toxicology. 2008;**46**:446-475. DOI: 10.1016/j.fct.2007.09.106

[4] Nieto G. Biological activities of three essential oils of the Lamiaceae Family. Medicine. 2017;**4**(3):63. DOI: 10.3390/medicines4030063

[5] Santos Silva L, Luz TRSA, de Mesquita JWC, Coutinho DF, do Amaral FMM, de Sousa Ribeiro MN, et al. Exploring the anticancer properties of essential oils from family Lamiaceae. Food Review International. 2019;**35**(2):105-131. DOI: 10.1080/87559129.2018.1467443

[6] Arabacı T, Uzay G, Keleştemur U, Karaaslan MG, Balcıoğlu S, Ateş B. Cytotoxicity, radical scavenging, antioxidant properties and chemical composition of the essential oil of *Satureja cilicica* P.H. Davis from Turkey. Journal of Research in PharmacyJournal of Research in Pharmacy. 2017;**21**(3):500-505. DOI: 10.12991/marupj.311814

[7] Yousefzadi M, Riahi-Madvar A, Hadian J, Rezaee F, Rafiee R. *In vitro* cytotoxic and antimicrobial activity of essential oil from *Satureja sahendica*. Toxicological and Environmental Chemistry. 2012;**94**(9):1735-1745. DOI: 10.1080/02772248.2012.728606

[8] Sadeghi I, Yousefzadi M, Behmanesh M, Sharifi M, Moradi A. In vitro cytotoxic and antimicrobial activity of essential oil from *Satureja Intermedia*. Iranian Red Crescent Medical Journal. 2013;**15**:70-74. DOI: 10.5812/ircmj.4989

[9] Sharifi-Rad J, Sharifi-Rad M, Hoseini-Alfatemi SM, Iriti M, Sharifi-Rad M, Sharifi-Rad M. Composition, cytotoxic and antimicrobial activities of *Satureja intermedia* CA Mey essential oil. International Journal of Molecular Sciences. 2015;**16**(8):17812-17825. DOI: 10.3390/ijms160817812

[10] Yousefzadi M, Riahi-Madvar A, Hadian J, Rezaee F, Rafiee R, Biniaz M. Toxicity of essential oil of *Satureja khuzistanica*: In vitro cytotoxicity and anti-microbial activity. Journal of Immunotoxicology. 2014;**11**(1):50-55. DOI: 10.3109/1547691X.2013.789939

[11] Kundaković T, Stanojković T, Kolundzija B, Marković S, Sukilović B, Milenković M, et al. Cytotoxicity and antimicrobial activity of the essential oil from *Satureja montana* subsp. pisidica (Lamiaceae). Natural Product Communications. 2014;**9**(4):569-572. DOI: europepmc.org/abstract/med/24868886

[12] Mohammadpour G, Tahmasbpour R, Noureini S, Tahmasbpour E, Bagherpour G. In vitro antimicrobial and cytotoxicity assays of *Satureja bakhtiarica* and *Zataria multiflora* essential oils. American Journal of Phytomedicine and Clinical Therapeutics. 2015;**3**(6):502-511. DOI: index.php/AJPCT/issue/view/35

[13] Sharifi-Rad J, Ayatollahi SA, Varoni EM, Salehi B, Kobarfard F, Sharifi-Rad M, et al. Chemical composition and functional properties of essential oils from *Nepeta Schiraziana* Boiss. Farmácia. 2017;**65**(5):802-812. DOI: 201705/issue52017art24.html

[14] Skorić M, Gligorijević N, Čavić M, Todorović S, Janković R, Ristić M, et al.

Cytotoxic activity of *Nepeta rtanjensis* Diklić & Milojević essential oil and its mode of action. Industrial Crops and Products. 2017;**100**:163-170. DOI: 10.1016/j.indcrop.2017.02.027

[15] Shakeria A, Khakdanb F, Soheilic V, Sahebkard A, Shaddelf R, Asilig J. Volatile composition, antimicrobial, cytotoxic and antioxidant evaluation of the essential oil from *Nepeta sintenisii* Bornm. Industrial Crops and Products. 2016;**84**:224-229. DOI: 10.1016/j.indcrop.2015.12.030

[16] Kahkeshani N, Razzaghirad Y, Ostad SN, Hadjiakhoondi A, Shams Ardekani MR, Hajimehdipoor H, et al. Cytotoxic, acetylcholinesterase inhibitor and antioxidant activity of *Nepeta menthoides* Boiss & Buhse essential oil. Journal of Essential Oil Bearing Plants. 2014;**17**(4):544-552. DOI: 10.1080/0972060X.2014.929040

[17] Tefiani C, Riazi A, Youcefi F, Aazza S, Gago C, Faleiro M, et al. *Ammoides pusilla* (Apiaceae) and Thymus munbyanus (Lamiaceae) from Algeria essential oils: Chemical composition, antimicrobial, antioxidant and antiproliferative activities. Journal of Essential Oil Research. 2015;**27**(2):131-139. DOI: 10.1080/10412905.2015.1006739

[18] Bendif H, Boudjeniba M, Miara MD, Biqiku L, Bramucci M, Lupidi G, et al. Essential oil of *Thymus munbyanus* subsp. *coloratus* from Algeria: Chemotypification and *in vitro* biological activities. Chemistry & Biodiversity. 2017;**14**(e1600299):1-19. DOI: 10.1002/cbdv.201600299

[19] Fekrazad R, Afzali M, Pasban-Aliabadi H, Esmaeili-Mahani S, Aminizadeh M, Mostafavi A. Cytotoxic effect of *Thymus caramanicus* Jalas on human oral epidermoid carcinoma KB cells. Brazilian Dental Journal. 2017;**28**(1):72-77. DOI: 10.1590/0103-6440201700737

[20] Hassan HM, Mina SA, Bishr MM, Khalik SMA. Influence of foliar spray of ethephon and water stress on the essential oil composition and impact on the cytotoxic activity of *Thymus vulgaris* aerial parts. Natural Product Research. 2018:1-4. DOI: 10.1080/14786419.2018.1460843

[21] Liu K, Zhu Q, Zhang J, Xu J, Wang X. Chemical composition and biological activities of the essential oil of *Mentha spicata* Lamiaceae. Advances in Materials Research. 2012;**524-527**:2269-2272. DOI: 10.4028/www.scientific.net/AMR.524-527.2269

[22] Miller AB, Cates RG, O'Neill K, Fuentes Soria JA, Espinoza LV, Alegre BF, et al. Evaluation of essential oils from 22 Guatemalan medicinal plants for *in vitro* activity against cancer and established cell lines. Journal of Medicinal Plants Research. 2018;**12**(3):42-49. DOI: 10.5897/JMPR2017.6528

[23] Nikolić M, Jovanović KK, Marković T, Marković D, Gligorijević N, Radulović S, et al. Chemical composition, antimicrobial, and cytotoxic properties of five Lamiaceae essential oils. Industrial Crops and Products. 2014;**61**:225-232. DOI: 10.1016/j.indcrop.2014.07.011

[24] Kathirvel P, Ravi S. Chemical composition of the essential oil from basil (*Ocimum basilicum* Linn.) and its *in vitro* cytotoxicity against HeLa and HEp-2 human cancer cell lines and NIH 3T3 mouse embryonic fibroblasts. Natural Product Research. 2012;**26**(12):1112-1118. DOI: 10.1080/14786419.2010.545357

[25] Mahmoud G. Biological effects, antioxidant and anticancer activities of marigold and basil essential oils. Journal of Medicinal Plant Research. 2013;**10**: 561-572. DOI: 10.5897/JMPR12.350

[26] Selvi MT, Thirugnanasampandan R, Sundarammal S. Antioxidant and

cytotoxic activities of essential oil of Ocimum canum Sims. From India. Journal of Saudi Chemical Society. 2015;**19**(1):97-100. DOI: 10.1016/j.jscs.2011.12.026

[27] De Lima VT, Vieira MC, Kassuya CAL, Cardoso CAL, Alves JM, Foglio MA, et al. Chemical composition and free radical-scavenging, anticancer and anti-inflammatory activities of the essential oil from *Ocimum kilimandscharicum*. Phytomedicine. 2014;**21**(11):1298-1302. DOI: 10.1016/j.phymed.2014.07.004

[28] Russo A, Formisano C, Rigano D, Senatore F, Bruno M. Chemical composition and anticancer activity of essential oils of Mediterranean sage (*Salvia officinalis* L.) grown in different environmental conditions. Food and Chemical Toxicology. 2013;**55**:42-47. DOI: 10.1016/j.fct.2012.12.036

[29] Eftekhari M, Shams Ardekani MR, Amini M, Akbarzadeh T, Safavi M, Razkenari EK, et al. Biological activities of the essential oil and total extract of *Salvia macrosiphon* Boiss. Journal of Basic and Clinical Pharmacy. 2017;**8**:82-86. Available from: https://www.jbclinpharm.org/articles/biological-activities-of-the-essential-oil-and-total-extract-of-salvia-macrosiphon-boiss.html#a1

[30] Donadu MG, Usai D, Mazzarello V, Molicotti P, Cannas S, Bellardi MG, et al. Change in Caco-2 cells following treatment with various lavender essential oils. Natural Product Research. 2017;**31**(18):2203-2206. DOI: 10.1080/14786419.2017.1280489

[31] Mantovani LLA, Vieira GPG, Cunha WR, Groppob M, Santos RA, Rodrigues V, et al. Chemical composition, antischistosomal and cytotoxic effects of the essential oil of *Lavandula angustifolia* grows in southeastern Brazil. Revista Brasileira de Farmacognosia. 2013;**23**:877-884. DOI: 10.1590/S0102-695X2 013000600004

[32] Zkan A, Erdonğan A. Comparative evaluation of antioxidant and anticancer activity of essential oil from *Origanum onites* (Lamiaceae) and its two major phenolic components. Turkish Journal of Biology. 2011;**35**:735-742. DOI: 10.3906/biy-1011-170

[33] Hussain AI, Anwar F, Rasheed S, Nigam PS, Janneh O, Sarker SD. Composition, antioxidant and chemotherapeutic properties of the essential oils from two *Origanum* species growing in Pakistan. Brazilian Journal of Pharmacognosy. 2011;**521**(6):943-952. DOI: 10.1590/S0102-695X2011005000165

[34] Grondona E, Gatti G, López AG, Sánchez LR, Rivero V, Pessah O, et al. Bio-efficacy of the essential oil of oregano (*Origanum vulgare* Lamiaceae. Ssp. Hirtum). Plant Foods for Human Nutrition. 2014;**69**(4):351-357. DOI: 10.1007/s11130-014-0441-x

[35] Oliveira PFD, Alves JM, Damasceno JL, Oliveira RAM, Júnior HD, Crotti AEM, et al. Cytotoxicity screening of essential oils in cancer cell lines. Revista Brasileira de Farmácia. 2015;**25**(2):183-188. DOI: 10.1016/j.bjp.2015.02.009

[36] Gazim ZC, Rodrigues F, Amorin ACL, Rezende CMD, Soković M, Tešević V, et al. New natural diterpene-type abietane from *Tetradenia riparia* essential oil with cytotoxic and antioxidant activities. Molecules. 2014;**19**(1):514-524. DOI: 10.3390/molecules19010514

[37] Venditti A, Frezza C, Maggi F, Lupidi G, Bramucci M, Quassinti L, et al. Phytochemistry, micromorphology and bioactivities of *Ajuga chamaepitys* (L.) Schreb. (Lamiaceae, Ajugoideae): Two new harpagide derivatives and an unusual iridoid glycosides pattern. Fitoterapia. 2016;**113**:35-43. DOI: 10.1016/j.fitote.2016.06.016

[38] Abu-Darwisha MS, Cabralc C, Gonçalvesc MJ, Cavaleiro C, Cruz MT,

Paolid M, et al. *Ziziphora tenuior* L. essential oil from Dana biosphere reserve (Southern Jordan); chemical characterization and assessment of biological activities. Journal of Ethnopharmacology. 2016;**194**:963-970. DOI: 10.1016/j.jep.2016.10.076

[39] Venditti A, Bianco A, Frezza C, Serafini M, Giacomello G, Giuliani C, et al. Secondary metabolites, glandular trichomes and biological activity of *Sideritis montana* L. subsp. Montana from Central Italy. Chemistry & Biodiversity. 2016;**13**:1380-1390. DOI: 10.1002/cbdv.201600082

[40] Venditti A, Bianco A, Quassinti L, Bramucci M, Lupidi G, Damiano S, et al. Phytochemical analysis, biological activity, and secretory structures of *Stachys annua* (L.) L. subsp. *annua* (Lamiaceae) from Central Italy. Chemistry & Biodiversity. 2015;**12**(8):1172-1183. DOI: 10.1002/cbdv.2014002759

[41] Thirugnanasampandan R, Ramya G, Gogulramnath M, Jayakumar R, Kanthimathi MS. Evaluation of cytotoxic, DNA protecting and LPS induced MMP-9 down regulation activities of *Plectranthus amboinicus* (Lour) Spreng. Essential oil. Pharmacological Reviews. 2015;**7**(1):32-36. DOI: 10.5530/pj.2015.1.3

[42] Saeidi M, Emami SA, Moshtaghi N, Malekzadeh-Shafaroudi S. Comparative volatile composition, antioxidant and cytotoxic evaluation of the essential oil of *Zhumeria majdae* from south of Iran. Iranian Journal of Basic Medical Sciences. 2019;**22**(1):80-85. DOI: 10.22038/ijbms.2018.20829.5418

[43] Zorzetto C, Sánchez-Mateo CC, Rabanal RM, Lupidi G, Bramucci M, Quassinti L, et al. Antioxidant activity and cytotoxicity on tumour cells of the essential oil from Cedronella canariensis var. canariensis (L.) Webb & Berthel. (Lamiaceae). Natural Product Research. 2015;**29**(17):1641-1649. DOI: 10.1080/14786419.2014.994213

[44] Awadh Ali NA, Chhetri BK, Dosoky NS, Shari K, Al-Fahad AJA, Wessjohann L, et al. Antimicrobial, antioxidant, and cytotoxic activities of *Ocimum forskolei* and *Teucrium yemense* (Lamiaceae) essential oils. Medicine. 2017;**4**(17):1-14. DOI: 101155/2019/8928306

[45] Han-Yu Z, Yang G, Peng-Xiang L. Chemical composition, antioxidant, antimicrobial and cytotoxic activities of essential oil from *Premna microphylla* Turczaninow. Molecules. 2017;**22**(381):1-11. DOI: 10.3390/molecules22030381

[46] Ashrafi B, Ramak P, Ezatpour B, Talei GR. Investigation on chemical composition, antimicrobial, antioxidant, and cytotoxic properties of essential oil from *Dracocephalum kotschyi* Boiss. African Journal of Traditional, Complementary and Alternative Medicines. 2017;**14**(3):209-217. DOI: 10.21010/ajtcam.v14i3.23

[47] Holbeck SL, Collins JM, Doroshow JH. Analysis of FDA-approved anti-cancer agents in the NCI60 panel of human tumor cell lines. Molecular Cancer Therapeutics. 2011;**9**(5):1451-1460. DOI: 10.1158/1535-7163.MCT-10-0106

[48] Nestorović J, Mišić D, Šiler B, Soković M, Glamočlija J, Ćirić A, et al. Nepetalactone content in shoot cultures of three endemic Nepeta species and the evaluation of their antimicrobial activity. Fitoterapia. 2010;**81**(6):621-626. DOI: 10.1016/j.fitote.2010.03.007

[49] JSTOR. Global Plants. Available from: https://plants.jstor.org/plants/browse Consulted 11-04-2019

Chapter 4

Cytotoxic Effect and Mechanisms from Some Plant-Derived Compounds in Breast Cancer

Elvia Pérez-Soto, Cynthia Carolina Estanislao-Gómez, David Guillermo Pérez-Ishiwara, Crisalde Ramirez-Celis and María del Consuelo Gómez-García

Abstract

Breast cancer (BrC) is a major health problem in women all around the world. A growing knowledge about these alterations and their associated molecular signaling pathways offers opportunities for therapeutic strategies; chemotherapy is one of the most utilized treatments; however, because of the adverse side effects and multidrug resistance that patients may present, there has been great advancement in search of new alternatives as the use of plant-derived natural compounds. This review describes information on the progress and development of cytotoxic compounds against BrC belonging to the families of flavonoids, terpenes, and alkaloids that through in vitro and in vivo studies have demonstrated to induce cellular death mainly through apoptosis, activating the intrinsic pathway. The in vitro IC_{50} and the in vivo EC_{50} dose-response relationship can vary depending on various factors, including the choice of cell line and/or the model used. Also, the association of some of these compounds with nanoparticles or paclitaxel with antibodies has clearly shown a potential improvement in its effect. The clinical studies that are being conducted with some of them show promising results; however, it is necessary to continue with the effort to develop new and more effective drugs against different types of BrC.

Keywords: breast cancer, cytotoxic agents, natural products, in vitro model, in vivo model, flavonoids, terpenoid, alkaloids, nanoparticles

1. Breast cancer (BrC)

Cancer is the uncontrolled and unregulated growth of cells that generally invade and destroy normal cells [1]. Breast cancer [BrC] is the deadliest malignancy in women worldwide and also an important public health problem being the second leading cause of cancer in women accounting for more than 626,679 deaths only in 2018 [2]. In many cases this disease has become fatal because of its multifactorial origin and also because it has a great number of exogenous and endogenous factors that can stimulate different pathways [3]. In early BrC, gene expression profiles are determined for hormone receptor (HR)-positive disease and human epidermal growth factor type 2 receptor (HER2) status which define if a patient is likely to receive systemic therapy and are therefore used to guide their treatment [4]. Approximately

60–70% of primary BrC cases express positive estrogen receptors (ER+) or positive progesterone receptors (PR+) or both and are hormone responsive. However, about 15–20% of BrC cases are in the category of triple-negative phenotype owing to their lack of ER, PR, and amplified HER2. Commonly, ER+ hormone-dependent BrCs have a better prognosis and are often responsive to antihormone therapy [4].

Because of these reasons, the survival rates for BrC have decreased significantly; however, there have been great advancements in new alternative therapies which not only are safer but are also more effective and inexpensive and have minimal side effects [5]. Therapeutic drugs derived from natural compounds have become of great interest since more than 75% of anticancer drugs were designed and developed from plant-derived natural ingredients which have been proven to have anticancer properties with novel mechanisms [6]. In the last 50 years, nearly 200 new chemical compounds have been approved to fight cancer, of which around 50% are molecules of unmodified natural products and their semisynthetic or synthetic derivatives that are safe and profitable [7, 8]. Small organic molecules such as terpenes, flavonoids, alkaloids, lignans, saponins, vitamins, minerals, glycosides, oils, and other secondary metabolites play a significant role in either the inhibition of proliferation, induction of apoptosis, or other mechanisms that may be altered [9, 10]. The structural diversity of natural products and their wide application in therapeutics have always been recognized by pharmaceutical industries [1].

This chapter summarizes the small novel organic molecules obtained from plants and their derivatives, some of which are on the market and others are found in preclinical studies with encouraging results. We also describe some interesting biotechnological associations between some compounds and nanoparticles or other molecules as antibodies that show a novel potential in the treatment of BrC.

2. In vitro models for studying plant-derived compounds in breast cancer

The evaluation of the therapeutic potential of novel plant-derived compounds or secondary metabolites, either pure compounds or the mixture of active constituents, can serve as chemotherapeutic agents in BrC. The biological models used for the development of new drugs include in vitro models using BrC cell lines and are divided into estrogen receptor positive (ER+, T47, MCF-7) and ER negative (ER-, MDA-MB-231, MDA-MB-453, SKBR3). MDA-MB-231 or triple-negative breast cancer cell (TNBC) line, estrogen negative (ER-) and progesterone negative (PR-), and HER- are known to be models for metastasis, which are more aggressive, containing a high potential to metastasize, and are unresponsive to antiestrogens [5, 8]. TNBC line is used to investigate the mechanism underlying migration and invasion. It is important to find cancer therapeutic compounds which possess multi-targeted and multifunctional potential with anti-metastasis activity [8, 11]. MCF-7 is the most used cell line with a great number of publications due to the presence of ER+ [9].

In vitro experiments have also been used in different studies, in order to characterize and identify compounds derived from extracts, essential oils, and other extractions. Trypan blue dye, MTT, sulforhodamine B, and lactic dehydrogenase assays constitute some of the most utilized assays used to evaluate the cytotoxic effect of essential oils and/or pure compounds in different cell lines of BrC. In order to characterize morphological changes, biochemical and molecular levels of cell death, proteins that are modified (expression and activation), gene regulation, migration, invasion, and cell division, among other changes, experiments such as staining with hematoxylin and eosin, Western blot, TUNEL, annexin V, qRT-PCR, scratch assay, and cell cycle assays are performed [12].

3. In vivo models for studying plant-derived compounds in breast cancer

Wide varieties of animal model systems are now available to investigate plant-derived compounds in different stages, such as cancer initiation, promotion progression, invasion, and metastasis. These models are also used to comprehend therapeutic response, which represents an essential step between in vitro systems and clinical studies [8, 13]. The in vivo models are also used to investigate the capability of plant formulation to induce an anti-BrC effect where it is sought to optimize dose, bioavailability, administration routes, and selective delivery and reduce toxic effects, among others [8, 14]. The two animal species that will be mentioned in this review are those involving mice and rats [14]; however, BrC mouse models are used in a variety of preclinical studies [13].

There are different types of in vivo models of BrC, such as cell line-derived xenografts (MDA-MB-231 line) that are implanted into immunocompromised animals (cell-derived xenografts, CDX). CDX models represent a relatively homogenous mass of transformed breast epithelial cells, and depending on where the cells are inoculated, they are classified as ectopic CDX (models advanced disease only, subcutaneous injection of human tumor cells), orthotopic CDX (in mammary gland/fat pad), metastatic CDX (following tail vein or intra-cardiac injection in specific sites, i.e., bone or lung), syngeneic (mouse tissue implanted to strain-matched host) or metastasis with syngeneic model (usually fast-growing tumors and microenvironment derive from the same species, i.e., 4T1 cells), and genetically engineered mouse models (GEMMs) to address early events of tumorigenesis [13]. Nonetheless, researchers need to consider the limitations of each model and the mechanism of action of the compound previously investigated in in vitro models.

4. Cytotoxicity of plant-derived compounds

Plants produce bioactive secondary metabolites such as flavonoids [15], terpenoids [1], alkaloids [16], tannins, and others, which have profusely been studied for BrC (1, 8). Here, we describe some terpenoid compounds such as *D*-limonene, camptothecin (CPT), paclitaxel, and ursolic acid (UA) and some flavonoids such as cynaroside, isoflavones as Biochanin A (BA) or ginsenoside R2, naringenin, and other novel cytotoxic compounds from different natural sources as shown in **Figure 1** and **Table 1**.

The anti-BrC activities of plant-derived compounds discussed in this chapter are taken from published articles that demonstrated an anti-BrC activity against specific cancer cell lines (see **Table 2**) and in vivo models (see **Table 3**) or clinical studies with their mechanism of action.

4.1 Terpenoids as cytotoxic compounds

Terpenoids are organic compounds derived from five-carbon units (isoprene) assembled and modified in different ways. The classification of terpenoids is based on the isoprene units which are commonly classified as monoterpenes (C10) and diterpenes (C20), i.e., paclitaxel, and triterpenes as ursolic acid [1]. Interestingly, essential oils are a rich and complex composition of monoterpenes with anti-BrC activity such as *Decatropis bicolor* essential oil (*DBEO*) [17].

4.1.1 D-limonene

D-limonene, (1-methyl-4-(1-methylethenyl-cyclohexene) a monocyclic monoterpene, with a molecular mass of 136.23 g/mol [18], is found in the peels of citrus

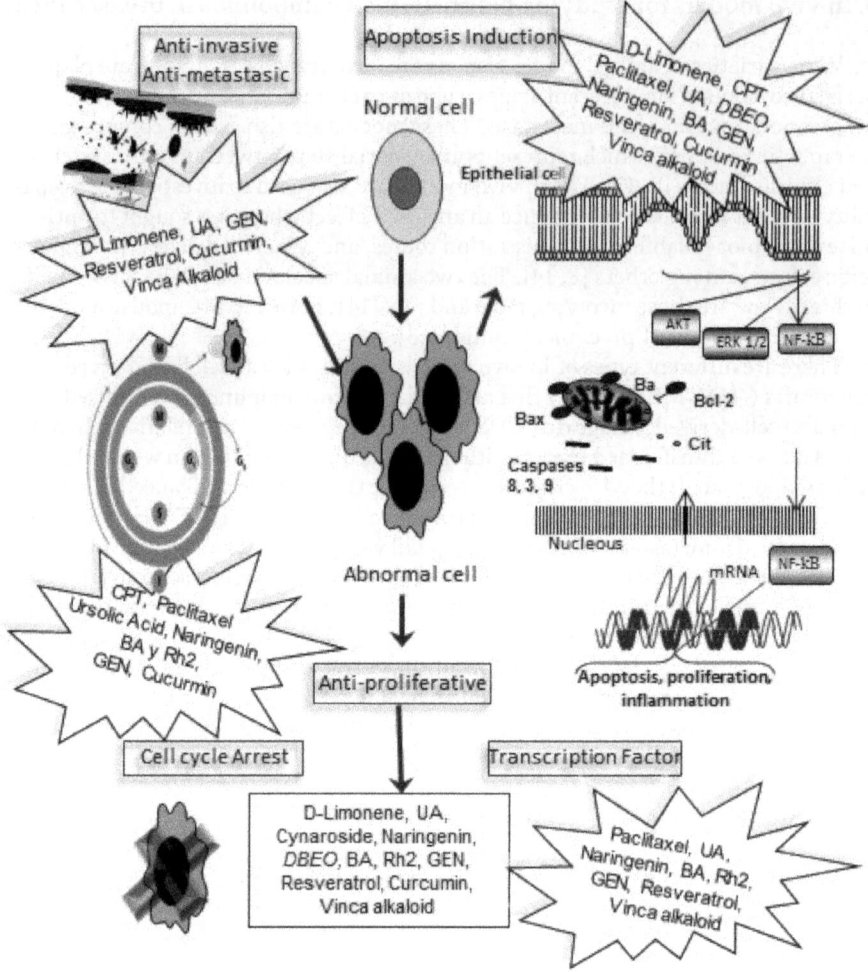

Figure 1.
Molecular targets of plant-derived compounds in BrC.

fruits [18–20]. The main mechanism described by *D*-limonene is the inhibition of the posttranslational isoprenylation of cell growth-regulatory proteins such as Ras, inducing cell death. It has also demonstrated to decrease the viability of cancer cells in a dose-dependent manner by inducing apoptotic cell death. It induced the activation of caspase-3 and caspase-9, PARP cleavage, and Bax protein and cytosolic release of cytochrome c from the mitochondria and through the attenuation of the expression of Bcl-2 protein, suggesting that *D*-limonene induces apoptosis via the mitochondrial pathway and through the suppression of the PI3K/AKT pathway [21, 22]. The interest in this compound as a potential cancer chemotherapeutic agent was stimulated by pronounced chemopreventive and chemotherapeutic efficacy in spontaneous and carcinogen-induced animal tumor models with little toxicity [19, 22]. In the in vivo models, it has been reported to exhibit various effects on several hallmarks of cancer (i.e., proliferation, apoptosis, inflammation) [23, 24]. 7,12-Dimethylbenz(a)anthracene (DMBA) and *N*-methyl-*N*-nitrosourea (MNU) induced mammary carcinogenesis in rats and induced regression of carcinomas [24–26]. Dietary feeding of *D*-limonene also inhibited the development of Ras oncogene in mammary carcinomas in rats [25].

Source	Compound	Study type	Concentration	Ref
Apples, herbs and spices including rosemary	Ursolic acid (UA)	MCF-7, MDA-MB-231	221.39 µg/ml 239.47 µg/ml	[33]
Apiaceae family, *Cuminum cyminum*	Cynaroside	MCF-7	IC_{50}:3.98 µg/ml	[42]
Soybeans, soy foods, legumes	Biochanin (BA)	MCF-7, MDA-MB-231	63.76 µm and 59.76 µm, respectively	[44]
Soybeans, soy foods, legumes	Ginsenoside (Rh2)	MCF-7, MDA-MB-231	57.53 µm and 52.53 µm, respectively	[44]
Soybeans, soy foods, legumes	Ginsenoside + biochanin	MDA-MB-231 MCF-7	27.68, 25.41 µm; 25.2 µm, and 22.75 µm	[44]
Tomatoes (*Solanum lycopersicum*), citrus fruits and grapes	Naringenin	MDA-MB-231	40 µg/ml	[43]
Soy products	Genistein (GEN)	MCF-7, MDA-MB-231 /ERβ1	100 µm	[48]
Tomatoes (*Solanum lycopersicum*), other red fruits	Lycopene (LYC)	MDA-MB-231 MCF-7	≥1.25 µm to 5 µl in TNBC. 50 µm	[11, 12]
LYC incorporated biopolymeric nanoparticles with whey protein isolate	Lycopene (LYC-WPI-NPs)	MCF-7	25–50 µm/ml	[49]
A derivative from D-limonene	Perillyl alcohol a hydroxylated product of D-limonene	KPL-1, MCF-7, MKL-F, MDA-MB-231	500 µm	[26]
Taxus brevifolia	Paclitaxel	MCF-7 T47-D, MBA-MB-231, MDA-MB-435	100–500 nm	[28]
Taxus brevifolia	Paclitaxel-loaded nanospheres	MDA-MB-435, ZR.75.1	0.06–0.6 ng/ml	[50]
Grapes, wine, nuts, berries	Resveratrol	MCF-7	10–150 µm	[51]
Camptotheca accuminata	Camptothecin	MDA-MB-231 MCF-7	100 nm IC_{50}:0.65 nm	[52, 53]
Curcuma longa	Curcumin	MCF-7 MCF-7 MDA-MB-231	IC_{50}: 29 µg/ml IC_{50}: 35 µm IC_{50}: 30 µm	[54, 55]
Vinca alkaloids	Vincristine	MCF-7, HeLa	IC_{50}: 170 and 50 nmol/L	[56]

Table 1.
Cytotoxic effect of plant-derived compounds in in vitro models of BrC.

4.1.2 Paclitaxel

Paclitaxel is a complex diterpene, with a molecular structure of $C_{47}H_{51}NO_{14}$ and a molecular mass of 853.91 g/mol [18]. This compound induces mitotic arrest and also apoptosis by activating extrinsic or intrinsic pathway. In MCF-7 cells it decreased levels of Bcl-2 protein and increased proapoptotic proteins such as Bax, cytochrome c, caspase-9, and caspase-3 [27, 28]. Likewise, it has also been reported

Compound	Study type	Dose and activity	Ref
D-Limonene	DMBA and NMU-induced mammary carcinogenesis in rats	10% of limonene diet. Induced complete regression of primary rat mammary tumors and prevented the development of secondary tumors	[24]
Perillyl alcohol a hydroxylated product of D-limonene	Mammary rat tumor induced with KPL-1 cells	75 mg/kg. Suppressed orthotopically transplanted KPL-1 tumor cell growth and regional lymph node metastasis in a nude mouse system	[26]
Paclitaxel-encapsulated liposomes	DMBA mammary tumor	20 mg/kg. In combination with 500 mg/kg of *Eruca sativa* extract reduced NF-κB, COX-2 and Bcl-2 gene expression	[97]
Paclitaxel-loaded nanospheres	Tumor xenograft model in mice	5–50 mg/kg. Showed an equivalent antitumor efficacy to the clinical formulation and provided a superior safety and improved tolerability to higher paclitaxel doses	[50]
Resveratrol	DMBA induced mammary cancer in rats estrogen-induced breast carcinoma in rats	100 μg/rat. Suppressed COX-2 and matrix metalloprotease-9 expression in the breast tumor. 50 mg. Inhibits breast carcinogenesis via induction of NRF2-mediated protective pathways	[67, 98]
Curcumin	MCF-7 xenografts mouse breast cancer model	100 mg/kg in combination with mitomycin 1–2 mg/kg. The combined treatment inhibited tumor growth, induced G1 arrest, and decreased cyclin D1, cyclin E, cyclin A, CDK2, and CDK4	[99]
Camptothecin	Mouse 4T1 breast tumor model	2 mg/kg in combination with 1.05 mg/kg of doxorubicin. Induced 70% of tumor volume reduction and caspase-3 induction	[100]

Table 2.
Compounds evaluated in in vivo model of BrC.

that the induction of apoptosis was independent of caspases [29]. The combination of paclitaxel with a compound that inhibits the mitotic slippage such as phenylethyl isothiocyanate (PEITC) induced apoptosis in MDA-MB-231 cells which are drug resistance [30]. Also, additional activities of taxol have been described including the effect on cell signaling and gene expression and activation of mitogen-activated protein kinases (MAPKs), Raf-1, and protein tyrosine kinases [29]. Paclitaxel has been approved by the FDA to be used alone, or in combination with other anticancer treatments, to treat BrC and other cancers [31, 32].

4.1.3 Ursolic acid

Ursolic acid (3-β-hydroxy-urs-12-en-28-oic acid) is a pentacyclic triterpenoid natural product and a member of the cyclosqualenoid family, commonly named as UA with a molecular structure of $C_{30}H_{48}C_3$ and a molecular mass of 456.7 g/mol [18]. UA is derived from diverse plants and fruits, such as rosemary (*Rosmarinus officinalis*), apple (*Malus domestica*), makino, cranberries (*Vaccinium macrocarpon*), pears (*Pyrus pyrifolia*), prunes (*Prunus domestica*), bearberries (*Arctostaphylos alpina*), loquat (*Eriobotrya japonica*), scotch heather (*Calluna vulgaris*), basil (*Ocimum sanctum*), and jamun (*Eugenia jambolana*) [9, 11]. UA posed different activity against BrC via several molecular mechanisms [7, 11, 33–35], and UA

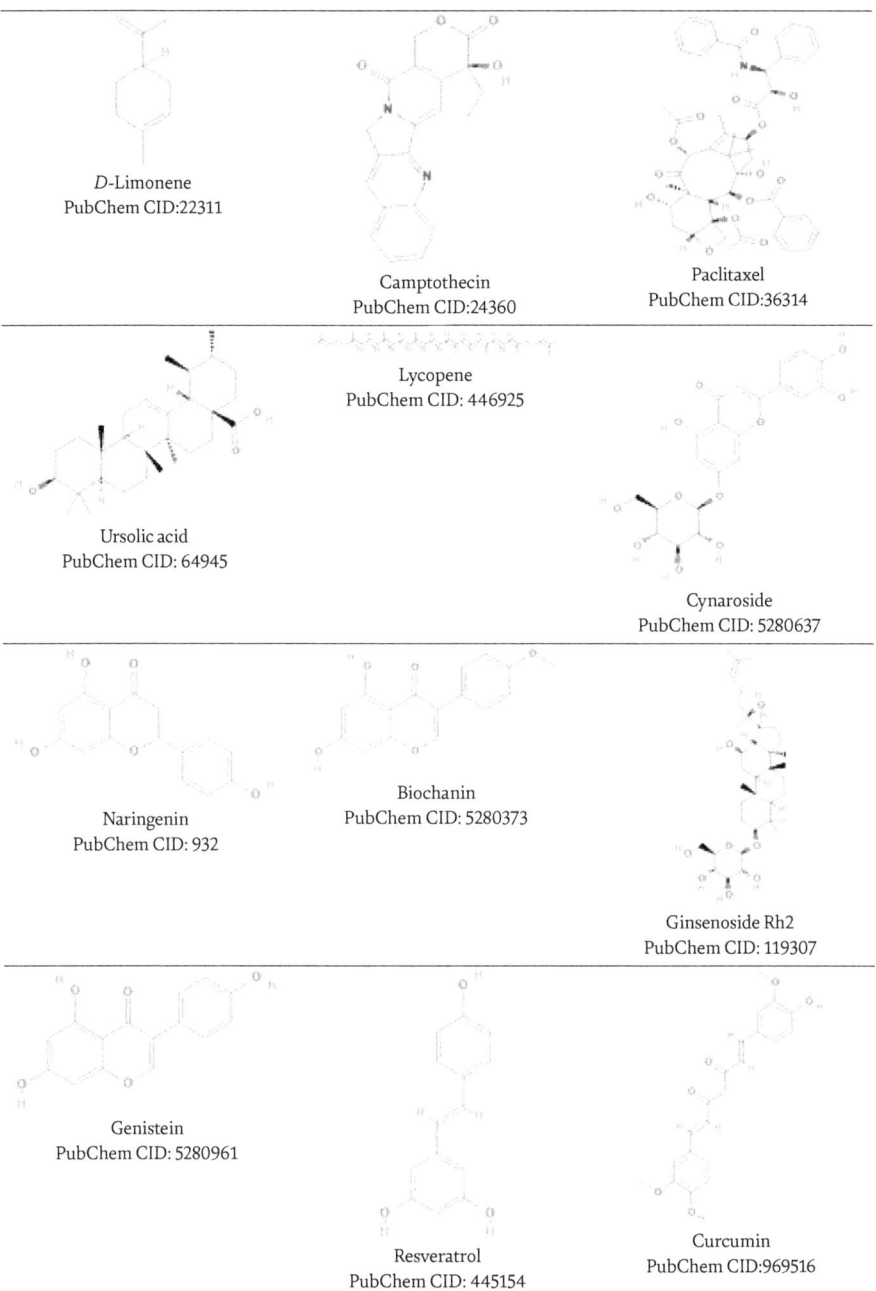

Table 3.
Structures of plant-derived compounds with potential effect in the BrC treatment.

is relatively nontoxic to normal cells [11]. Administration of UA demonstrates inhibitory efficacy against cell proliferation rate and induces apoptosis via both the mitochondrial death pathway (cleavage of caspase-9, caspase-3, and PARP, Bax upregulation and Bcl-2 downregulation, release of cytochrome c to the cytosol, decreased mitochondrial membrane potential) and extrinsic death receptor-dependent pathway (Fas receptor) in MDA-MB-231 cells [9, 11]. The treatment of BrC cells with UA induced changes in glycolytic pathway leading to cytotoxic autophagy, also at low doses (5–20 μm) caused a G0/G1 cell cycle arrest, increased p21 levels, oxidative stress, and DNA damage [36]. UA has been demonstrated to exhibit strong anti-BrC potential by inducing cell cycle arrest and inhibition of proliferation, angiogenesis, and metastasis in both in vitro and in vivo models [7, 11, 33–35]. Finally, UA inhibited BrC growth by inducing cell death via the inhibition of inflammatory responses through the NF-κB, PI3K/AKT signaling pathways [9, 33]. Therefore, UA could be used as a potential anti-BrC strategy in clinical studies.

4.1.4 Lycopene alone

Lycopene (LYC) (trans-lycopene) is a terpene assembled from eight isoprene units and is a rich antioxidant compound, a major carotenoid present in tomatoes (*Solanum lycopersicum*), apricots, red oranges, pink grapefruit, watermelon, rose hips, guava, vegetables, and photosynthetic algae [37]. LYC has a molecular structure of $C_{40}H_{56}$ and a molecular mass of 536.888 g/mol [18]. LYC is a compound that has displayed antiproliferative, anti-migration, anti-invasive, anti-metastatic, and antioxidant characteristics in numerous in vitro and in vivo studies in BrC [9, 37–39]. Also, LYC induces apoptosis and activates caspase-9 enzyme in human BrC cells [9]. Finally, LYC has inhibited the multiplication of cancer cells by arresting cell cycle at different phases (G1, S, and M phases) and by sustained activation of the ERK½ with suppression of cyclin D1 and upregulation of p21 [39]. Other mechanism of action of LYC is through the inhibition of IκBα phosphorylation and decrease in the expression of NF-κB [40].

4.1.5 Decatropis bicolor essential oil: a mixture of monoterpenes

Essential oils are a complex mixture of secondary metabolites such as monoterpenes that are responsible for their biological activity that includes anti-BrC effect. However, some studies suggested a synergistic activity of the compounds [17]. For example, DBEO was studied on MDA-MB-231 cells.

It had a cytotoxic effect with an IC_{50} of 53.81 μg/ml. It induced DNA fragmentation and apoptosis via intrinsic pathways due to the activation of Bax, caspase-9, and caspases-3, suggesting a synergistic activity of compounds present in the essential oil, such as 1,5-cyclooctadiene, 3-(methyl-2)propenyl, β-terpineol, 1-(3-methyl-cyclopent-2-enyl)-cyclohexene, *D*-limonene, pinene, and linalool [41].

4.2 Flavonoids as cytotoxic compounds

Flavonoids which are polyphenolic substances found in different plant-derived food are divided into flavones (cynaroside), flavonols, flavanones (naringenin), flavanols, isoflavones (genistein (GEN), biochanin A), anthocyanidins, and nonflavonoids [10]. Flavonoids have been reported to have an effect on BrC through numerous mechanisms such as antioxidant, anti-inflammatory, antiproliferative, cytotoxic, anti-angiogenic, and anti-metastatic effects in numerous in vitro and in vivo experiments in estrogen-dependent or estrogen-independent BrC [15, 37] (**Tables 1–3**).

4.2.1 Cynaroside

Cynaroside (luteolin-7-*O*-glucoside) is a glycosyloxyflavone or a glycoside form. It derives from luteolin. Cynaroside has a molecular structure of $C_{21}H_{20}O_{11}$ and a molecular mass of 448.38 g/mol [18]. Cynaroside is a constituent of the leaves of

Capsicum annuum (red pepper) and seeds and fruits of *Cuminum cyminum*, an old famous medicinal and culinary plant from the Apiaceae family. Currently, Goodarzi and collaborators demonstrated that luteolin-7-O-glucoside plays a significant role in cytotoxic effect of *C. cyminum* against MCF-7 cell line (IC_{50} of 3.98 μg/ml) and can be introduced as a candidate for chemopreventive and chemotherapeutic drugs [42]. More in vitro or in vivo studies are necessary to elucidate its mechanism of action.

4.2.2 Naringenin

Naringenin (4',5,7-trihydroxyflavanone) is a flavanone and member of 4'hydroxyflavanones; it has a molecular structure of $C_{15}H_{12}O_5$ and a molecular mass of 272.256 g/mol [18]. This bioflavonoid is a constituent of tomatoes, citrus fruits, and grapes. Naringenin is a phytoestrogen which is also an important anti-BrC, reported to be involved in decreasing the number of ER-α-positive cells by modulating p38 MAPK signaling pathway [9]. Recently, investigators reported that naringenin has antiproliferative effects by arresting the cell cycle at the G2 phase and caused an inhibitory effect on MDA-MB-231 cells via induction of apoptosis and inhibition of caspase-3 and caspase-9 activities [37, 43].

4.2.3 Biochanin and ginsenoside Rh2 as pure compounds or mixture

Biochanin or 4'-methylgenistein (B5,7-dihydroxy-4'-methoxyisoflavone) is an O-methylated isoflavone that is isolated from red clover *Trifolium pratense* and the root of *Astragalus membranaceus*, a traditional Chinese herbal medicine. BA has a molecular structure of $C_{16}H_{12}O_5$ and a molecular mass of 284.267 g/mol [18, 44]. The phytoestrogen BA caused antiproliferative activity by stabilizing and activating p53 through the upregulated expression of phospho-p53, phospho-p38, and p-ASK1 and downregulated expression of TRAF2 in MDA-MB-231 and MCF-7 cells [44] and apoptosis through upregulated expression of mRNA levels of ER-α, Bcl-2, and miR-375 in ER+ BrC cells, that is to say T47D and MCF-7 [37, 44, 45].

Also, BA stopped cell growth by blocking the activity of aromatase enzyme which is encoded by the gene CYP19 [5]. On the other hand, ginsenoside Rh2 (protopanaxadiol-type) is the major type of saponin ginsenoside that is separated from *Panax ginseng* and other species. Rh2 has a molecular structure of $C_{36}H_{62}O_8$ and a molecular mass of 622.884 g/mol [18, 44]. Rh2 exhibits antitumor activity in ER+(MCF-7) and ER-(MDA-MB-231). However, Ren and collaborators determined that BA plus Rh2 synergistically enhanced the antiproliferative effect in both BrC cells, with decreased EC_{50} values of both the compounds and a mechanism through the stabilization and activation of p53, p38, and ASK1 proteins (**Table 1**) [44].

4.2.4 Genistein

Genistein (4',5,7-trihydroxyisoflavone) is an isoflavonoid derived from soy products [46]. It has a molecular structure of $C_{15}H_{10}O_5$ and a molecular mass of 270.24 g/mol [18]. This agent has an antineoplastic effect in BrC [47]. GEN inhibits the growth of MDA-MB-231 cells by altering the phosphorylation of proteins included in cell cycle regulation and DNA damage response predominantly, and GEN induced apoptosis via the upregulation of Bax and p21WAF1 proteins in MDA-MB-231 cells and downregulating the expression of caspase-3 [5, 47]. In a recent study, GEN increases cell cycle arrest in G2/M phase in MDA-MB-231/ERβ1 cells, even though there is a high dose of GEN-arrested cells in G0/G1, just like in the MCF-7 cells. Thus, the combinatorial effect of GEN and overexpressed ERβ1 resulted in an active blockade of cell cycle progression and a dramatic inhibition of proliferation in vitro in MCF7 and MDA-MB-231 cells [48]. GEN could be a potential therapeutic agent for ERβ1-positive cancer, which merits further clinical research in the future.

4.2.5 Resveratrol

Resveratrol (3,5,4'-trihydroxy-*trans*-stilbene) is a natural nonflavonoid polyphenol with a molecular formula of $C_{14}H_{12}O_3$ [18]. These compounds are isolated from more than 72 species of plants including peanuts, grapes, mulberries, bilberries, and blueberries [9].

Numerous in vitro studies have shown that resveratrol has multiple anticancer effects, which protect the cells against both tumor initiation and cancer progression pathway [9, 57]. The activity of this compound was described in hormone-dependent or non-hormone-dependent BrC cells, in which it was found to induce apoptosis by intrinsic pathway through the upregulation of Bax, Bak, caspase-3, p53, and Akt pathway in different breast cancer cell lines and downregulated Bcl-2 and NF-kB and VEGF [51, 58–62]. Also, it can induce the extrinsic pathway through the expression of CD95 receptor [63]. A cell surface resveratrol receptor on the extracellular domain of heterodimeric αVβ3-integrin in MCF-7 human BrC cells induces extracellular-regulated kinases 1 and 2 (ERK1/2) and serine-15-p53-dependent phosphorylation leading to a p53-dependent apoptosis [57]. In several in vivo models, resveratrol supplementation was shown to decrease the incidence of mammary tumor formation, tumor volume, metastasis, and induced apoptosis [64–66]. The effect of resveratrol demonstrated lower tumor growth, decreased angiogenesis, and increased apoptotic index in ERα− and ERβ+ [62]. Also, the following can suppress mammary carcinogenesis in rats induced by DMBA: dietary administration of resveratrol (10 ppm), downregulation of NF-kB, cyclooxygenase-2 and matrix metalloprotease-9 expression in the breast tumor, and decreased tumor incidence [67, 68].

The effect of resveratrol in cancer patients has been investigated in a few clinical trials. The first clinical trial dealing with resveratrol and cancer was performed by Nguyen and collaborators in 2009, through the administration of 0.07 mg/day of resveratrol which resulted in the reduction of Wnt target gene expression, indicating that it may play a beneficial role in the prevention of cancer. These clinical trials have demonstrated resveratrol to be a promising therapeutic and chemopreventive agent [64, 69, 70].

4.2.6 Curcumin

Curcumin (1,7-bis(4-hydroxy-3-methoxyphenyl)-1,6-heptadiene-3,5-dione) is an orange-yellow component of turmeric or curry powder; it is a polyphenol natural product isolated from the rhizome of *Curcuma longa* [9, 71]. Curcumin has antiproliferative and proapoptotic effects against a variety of cancer cells in vitro. The anticancer effects observed by activating intrinsic apoptotic pathway by interacting with reactive oxygen species can release cytochrome C; upregulate caspase-9, caspase-3, Bax, and Bad; downregulate Bcl-2 antiapoptotic proteins; and induce DNA fragmentation in different BrC cell lines [72–75]. Also, it was found that curcumin inhibits the expression of Ki-67, proliferating cell nuclear antigen (PCNA), p53, and VEGF in BrC cells [54, 76]. Curcumin prevents carcinogen-induced cancers in rodents [77]. Banerjee et al. [79] reported that curcumin-induced G2/M arrest and apoptosis inhibited cell proliferation in MCF-7 cells, leading to an accumulation in the G1 phase, and suppressed the expression of zeste homolog 2 (EZH2) gene via MAPK pathway [78, 79].

4.3 Alkaloids as cytotoxic compounds

Alkaloids are a highly diverse group of compounds containing an organic nitrogen atom and a ring structure. Additionally, in most alkaloids the nitrogen atom is located inside the heterocyclic ring structure, which gives them a great biological diversity [16]. The structural diversity of this family is due to the wide number of amino acids used as building blocks [80]. Indeed, the peptide ring that they contain has one or more of its hydrogen atoms replaced with various alkyl radicals, most of which contain oxygen [81, 82]. Consequently, alkaloids can interact with a wide spectrum of molecules. They have a wide distribution in the plant kingdom and are a chemically heterogeneous group of ~17,000 molecules which have displayed pronounced biological and pharmacological activities. Furthermore, several alkaloids exhibit significant biological activities, with their unlimited supply of variable structures as well as their relatively low toxicity and well-documented stability; therefore, alkaloids are being used for their anticancer activity against various cancers [83].

4.3.1 Camptothecin

Camptothecin is a monoterpene indole alkaloid that consists of five rings [18], commonly named as CPT with a molecular structure of $C_{20}H_{16}N_2C_4$ and a molecular mass of 348.35 g/mol [18]. The antitumor activity of this compound is mainly due to its interaction with topoisomerase I (Top1), an enzyme involved in the regulation of DNA topology during replication, recombination, and transcription. It induces cell death by stabilizing a covalent complex between DNA topoisomerase I and the nicked DNA, leading to a DNA lesion [84–87].

CPT antitumoral activity has been reported in different cancer cell lines. Low doses of this compound lead to cell cycle arrest in the G2/M phase and inhibit DNA synthesis but at higher doses cause cell cycle arrest in S phase [52]. Also, the expression of some genes as c-Myc, Bax, BFL1, Bak, pRb2, c-Jun, and Jun-B was upregulated, and Cdk4, cyclin B1, Wee1, CRAF1, and DP1 were downregulated. Among these derivatives, camptothecin-20(s)-*O*-(2-pyrazolyl-1)acetic ester exhibited antitumor activity which demonstrated cytotoxicity, DNA fragmentation, and apoptosis toward MCF-7 cell line [53]. Also, in different studies in vivo, where it was delivered using an intralipid formulation through intramuscular (IM) route, CPT showed nearly 100% growth inhibition and regression in the colon, lung, breast, stomach, and ovary and malignant melanoma xenografts [88, 89].

4.3.2 Vinca alkaloids: vinblastine, vincristine, and vinorelbine

There are some vinca alkaloids in clinical use such as vinblastine, vinorelbine, and vincristine. Many alkaloids have poisonous characteristics but also have physiological effects that make them useful as medications. The oldest group of the plant alkaloids used to treat cancer is the vinca alkaloids. They have a dimeric chemical structure composed of two basic multi-ringed units, an indole nucleus (catharanthine) and a dihydroindole nucleus (vindoline), joined together with other complex systems. Structurally, vincristine and vinblastine are identical except for a single substitution on the vindoline nucleus, where vincristine and vinblastine possess formyl and methyl groups, respectively [90, 91] (**Table 2**). The main mechanisms of vinca alkaloid cytotoxicity is due to their interactions with tubulin and disruption of microtubule function, particularly of microtubules comprising the mitotic spindle apparatus, directly causing metaphase arrest. The disturbing effects occur at drug concentrations below those that decrease microtubule mass [91, 92]. Also, disorganization of the microtubule structure provokes the induction of tumor suppressor gene p53 and activation/inactivation of several protein kinases involved in key signaling pathways, including p21, WAF1/CIP1, Ras/Raf, and PKC/PKA, the apoptosis inhibitor Bcl2 and induction of Bax triggering the process of apoptosis in the cell [93]. These alkaloids demonstrated significant antitumor activity in patients with BrC. Also, xenograft mice models were used to evaluate low doses of vinblastine, which resulted in significant but transient xenograft regression, diminishing tumor vascularity, and direct inhibition of angiogenesis. Also, a combination therapy resulted in full and sustained regressions of large established tumors, without an ensuing increase in host toxicity or any signs of acquired drug resistance during treatment [94].

The risk of side effects and multidrug resistance limited the development of vinca alkaloids for clinical applications. To solve these problems, researchers have developed numerous strategies, such as using liposome-entrapped drugs, chemically modified drugs, and polymeric packaging drugs, to reduce the toxicity and enhance the therapeutic efficiency of vinca alkaloids. Many liposome products are still being tested in clinical trials. Another strategy for reducing chemotherapeutic toxicity involves using chemically modified drugs [95, 96].

5. Biotechnological and clinical advances of plant-derived compounds in breast cancer

Nanotechnology has been found to potentially improve current methods for disease, diagnosis, disease-state imaging, and treatment in BrC.

Targeted nanoparticle drug delivery is intended to reduce the side effects of anticancer drugs with both decreasing consumption and treatment expenses, which are the major hurdles in conventional cancer treatment. These small entities can be used in combination with a variety of plant-derived compounds in BrC with a variety of formulations being developed, making them a desirable choice of drug formulation [8].

5.1 Use of phytochemical compounds coupled to nanoparticles

5.1.1 Lycopene with nanoparticles

Recently, Jain and collaborators designed and synthesized LYC incorporated with biopolymeric nanoparticles with whey protein isolate nanoparticles (WPI NPs) with encouraging results in the compatibility of LYC-WPI-NPs over plain LYC as an optimum delivery system in vitro because encapsulation process did not affect its anticancer activity even in in vivo tumor model of DMBA where ~57% of LYC group of animals developed tumor compared with ~29% of LYC-WPI-NPs. The new formulation (LYC-WPI-NPs) posed higher cytotoxicity and cellular uptake efficacy as compared to the plain LYC in MCF-7 cells. Antitumoral effect of LYC-WPI-NPs and survival data indicate that proposed formulation strategy is a novel approach for the synchronized delivery of bioactive compound, leading to increased bioavailability, therapeutic efficacy, and safety profiling because of improvement in animal survival (100%), in contrast to animals free of LYC (66.67%) and negative control group (16.67%). This will certainly open new avenues to explore cancer treatment [49].

5.1.2 Paclitaxel with nanoparticles

As a strongly hydrophobic drug, it requires suitable delivery vehicles to effectively distribute into tumor tissues. For efficient distribution of this hydrophobic anticancer drug, paclitaxel is currently formulated and administered to patients via polyethoxylated castor oil (Cremophor EL, CrEL), but it is reported as causing hypersensitivity reactions and neurotoxicity [101]. To date, paclitaxel albumin-bound nanoparticles (Abraxane®) have been approved by the FDA for the treatment of metastatic BrC and non-small cell lung cancer [8]. Nanoparticle-based delivery systems can take advantage of the enhanced permeability and retention (EPR) effect for passive tumor targeting; therefore, they can improve the therapeutic index and decrease the side effects of paclitaxel. In addition, there are a number of novel paclitaxel nanoparticle formulations in clinical trials [50, 101–104]. Nanoparticle-assisted chemotherapeutic drug delivery has been used because it enhances therapeutic effectiveness. Studies on metastatic BrC demonstrate the inhibition of metastasis by co-delivering chemotherapeutic agent paclitaxel and twist shRNA via complex nanoparticles [105].

5.1.3 Camptothecin with nanoparticles

Research have concentrated on the development of potential delivery system to increase the aqueous solubility, stability, and bioavailability as well as controlled delivery of camptothecin at or around cancer tissues. For that purpose nanoencapsulation of drugs in a biodegradable polymer has been reported to protect the drug in the core of the polymeric shell [106–108]. Camptothecin encapsulated in nanoparticles demonstrated antitumor activity in in vitro and in vivo models; in MCF-7 cells the IC50 was lower (0.23 μm) than the pure compound (0.57 μm) [106, 109].

5.1.4 Curcumin with nanoparticles

As other compounds, in order to increase photostability and enhance its anticancer activity against BrC cells, scientists have formulated the transferrin-mediated solid lipid nanoparticle, which enhances the anticancer effect of curcumin in BrC cells in vitro [110]. A polymer-drug conjugate called polycurcumins also has advantages of high drug-loading efficiency, fixed drug-loading contents, stabilized curcumin in their backbones, and tailored water solubility. The polycurcumins are cytotoxic to cancer cells, but a polyacetal-based polycurcumin is highly cytotoxic to MCF-7 cells. The effect of these polymers induced cell cycle arrest and apoptosis partially through the caspase-3-dependent pathway. In vivo, this polymer showed antitumor activity in SKOV-3 intraperitoneal xenograft tumor model [111].

5.2 Novel therapies: antibody-phytopharmaceutical conjugates in breast cancer

In recent years, natural products and their derivatives have been among the major sources of drugs for the treatment of cancer as well as nanoparticles or antibodies. Furthermore, new treatments for different cases of BrC are necessary; this involves linking each cytotoxic drug concerned with a mAb by a linker group to produce a tripartite drug called an "antibody-drug conjugate" (ADC). A means of selective delivery of highly cytotoxic natural products as "prodrugs" to tumor cells has proven necessary in order to reduce off-target effects and increase therapeutic outcomes [8, 112].

5.2.1 Plant natural products as components of development ADCs: nab-paclitaxel or Abraxane®

The plant-derived compounds are secondary metabolites that have a different mechanism of action; although all of them are cytotoxic for BrC cells, new tools are being sought to increase their effectiveness, with less toxic effects. Also, incorporation of paclitaxel in liposomes can facilitate its delivery to cancer cells and eliminate the adverse reactions associated with the Cremophor EL vehicle. The lipid components of the liposomal formulation were nontoxic, but the intracellular paclitaxel levels were higher when MCF-7 cells were treated with the liposomal paclitaxel formulation; also, liposomal paclitaxel was as effective as conventional paclitaxel in inducing G2/M arrest after 1 day of treatment with 10 mmol/L, increasing the percentage of cells in this population from about 20% in cycling cells to over 60% after 7 days [104].

Abraxane® or nanoparticle albumin-bound paclitaxel (nab-paclitaxel) suspension demonstrated greater efficacy with less toxicity than docetaxel in metastatic BrC. This treatment has been approved to reduce toxicity and increased overall survival rates, compared to the parent compound [8]. Nab-paclitaxel is a neoadjuvant chemotherapy in HER2-negative BrC stages I, II, and III.

The recommended dose of Abraxane® is 260 mg/m^2 administered intravenously for 30 minutes, every 3 weeks. The results suggest that Abraxane® is effective in patients with highly proliferative cancers (81).

6. Conclusion

In nature, plants contain secondary metabolites, which have been used by humans to treat different diseases, since they have a complex diversity of chemical structures that have been specifically related to have anti-BrC activity in several preclinical studies with more than one mechanism of action; as a result, they can provide greater degree of efficacy. Several natural compounds are highlighted in this chapter, and their mechanism of action, synergistic action, nano-formulations, and future potentials are widely discussed, and due to the promising potential they represent, in fact, some of them are already used as treatment for BrC. However, it is necessary to have a greater diversity of drugs to be able to treat each one of the different tumors of BrC, since each BrC is different and many of these drugs may still induce several side effects and the development of mechanisms of resistance to drugs must be avoided. Subsequent from this review, we can conclude that although there are many compounds that have been characterized mainly in in vitro models and only around 10–20% of these were also evaluated in in vivo models and less than 10% are being evaluated already in clinical phases, it is essential to conduct more research on these compounds to learn their mechanism of action. Also, in their cellular, biochemical, and molecular levels, clinical effects as well as their genetic toxicities should be investigated sufficiently. Compounds that meet the eligibility criteria in these tests should be taken into clinical trial phase, and they may be administered in combination with other compounds or materials that make their pharmacological effect more efficient, make their arrival to the target site more selective, and guarantee their stability, bioavailability, pharmacokinetics, etc. In conclusion, addressing the study of these compounds in clinical phase is a pressing need.

Acknowledgements

This work was supported by the Secretaría de Investigación y Posgrado del Instituto Politécnico Nacional Grants SIP20170567 and SIP20196913. CRC is supported by CONACyT and BEIFI, IPN Fellowships.

Conflict of interest

The authors declare that they have no competing interests.

Author details

Elvia Pérez-Soto, Cynthia Carolina Estanislao-Gómez,
David Guillermo Pérez-Ishiwara, Crisalde Ramirez-Celis and
María del Consuelo Gómez-García*
Laboratorio de Biomedicina Molecular I, Programa Institucional de Biomedicina
Molecular, Escuela Nacional de Medicina y Homeopatía-Instituto Politécnico
Nacional, Ciudad de México, México

*Address all correspondence to: cgomezg@ipn.mx; consuelogg22@yahoo.com.mx

IntechOpen

© 2019 The Author(s). Licensee IntechOpen. This chapter is distributed under the terms of the Creative Commons Attribution License (http://creativecommons.org/licenses/by/3.0), which permits unrestricted use, distribution, and reproduction in any medium, provided the original work is properly cited.

References

[1] Prakash V. Terpenoids as cytotoxic compounds: A perspective. Pharmacognosy Reviews. 2018;**12**:166-176. Available from: http://www.phcogrev.com/text.asp?2018/12/24/166/243198

[2] Bray F, Ferlay J, Soerjomataram I, Siegel R, Torre L, Jemal A. Global cancer statistics 2018: GLOBOCAN estimates of incidence and mortality worldwide for 36 cancers in 185 countries. CA: A Cancer Journal for Clinicians. 2018;**68**(6):394-424. DOI: 10.3322/caac.21492

[3] Pavlova NN, Thompson Craig B. The emerging hallmarks of cancer metabolism. Cell Metabolism. 2016;**23**(1):27-47. DOI: 10.1016/j.cmet.2015.12.006

[4] Murphy C, Muscat A, Ashley D, Mukaro V, West L, Liao Y, et al. Tailored NEO adjuvant epirubicin, cyclophosphamide and nanoparticle albumin-bound paclitaxel for breast cancer: The phase II NEONAB trial—Clinical outcomes and molecular determinants of response. Plos One. 2019;**14**(2):1-20. DOI: 10.1371/journal.pone.0210891

[5] Mitra S, Dash R. Natural products for the management and prevention of breast cancer. Evidence-Based Complementary and Alternative Medicine. 2018;**2018**:1-24. DOI: 10.1155/2018/8324696

[6] Newman DJ, Cragg GM. Natural products as sources of new drugs from 1981 to 2014. Journal of Natural Products. 2016;**79**:629-661. DOI: 10.1021/acs.jnatprod.5b01055

[7] Iqbal J, Ahsan B, Ahmad R, Mahmood T, Kanwal S, Ali B, et al. Ursolic acid a promising candidate in the therapeutics of breast cancer: Current status and future implications. Biomedicine & Pharmacotherapy. 2018;**108**:752-756. DOI: 10.1016/j.biopha.2018.09.096

[8] Agarwal G, Carcache PB, Addo EM, Kinghorn AD. Current status and contemporary approaches to the discovery of antitumor agents from higher plants. Biotechnology Advances. 2019. DOI: 10.1016/j.biotechadv.2019.01.004

[9] Iqbal J, Ahsan B, Mahmood T, Ali B, Talha A, Kanwal S, et al. Potential phytocompounds for developing breast cancer therapeutics: Nature's healing touch. European Journal of Pharmacology. 2018;**827**:125-148. DOI: 10.1016/j.ejphar.2018.03.007

[10] Avtanski D, Poretsky L. Phyto-polyphenols as potential inhibitors of breast cancer metastasis. Molecular Medicine. 2018;**24**(1). DOI: 10.1186/s10020-018-0032-7

[11] Kim KH, Seo HS, Choi HS, Choi I, Shin YC, Ko S. Induction of apoptotic cell death by ursolic acid through mitochondrial death pathway and extrinsic death receptor pathway in MDA-MB-231 cells. Archives of Pharmacal Research. 2011;**34**(8):1363-1372. DOI: 10.1007/s12272-011-0817-5

[12] Tariq A, Sadia S, Pan K, Ullah I, Mussarat S, Sun F, et al. A systematic review on ethnomedicines of anti-cancer plants. Physical Therapy Research. 2017;**31**(2):202-264. DOI: 10.1002/ptr.5751

[13] Holen I, Speirs V, Morrissey B, Blyth K. *In vivo* models in breast cancer research: Progress, challenges and future directions. Disease Models & Mechanisms. 2017;**10**:359-371. DOI: 10.1242/dmm.028274

[14] Cekanova M. Animal models and therapeutic molecular targets of

cancer: Utility and limitations. Drug Design, Development and Therapy. 2014;**8**:1911-1922

[15] Sak K. Epidemiological evidences on dietary flavonoids and breast cancer risk: A narrative review. Asian Pacific Journal of Cancer Prevention. 2017;**18**(9):2309-2328

[16] Lu J-J, Bao J-L, Chen X-P, Huang M, Wang Y-T. Alkaloids isolated from natural herbs as the anticancer agents. Evidence-based Complementary and Alternative Medicine. 2012;**2012**:1-12. DOI: 10.1155/2012/485042

[17] Estanislao Gómez CC. PID and GGM. Biological activities of some essential oils from plants of Mexico. Journal of Complementary Medicine & Alternative Healthcare. 2017;**3**(3):3-6

[18] U.S. National Library of Medicine. Pub Chem Identifier [Internet]. 2019. Available from: https://pubchem.ncbi.nlm.nih.gov/compound/

[19] Erasto P, Viljoen A. Limonene—A review: Biosynthetic, ecological and pharmacological relevance. Natural Product Communications. 2008;**3**(7):1193-1199

[20] Malko MW, Wróblewska A, Chemical O. The importance of R-(+)-limonene as the raw material for organic syntheses and for organic industry. Chemik. 2016;**70**(4):193-202

[21] Jia S, Xi G, Zhang M, Chen Y, Lei BO, Dong X, et al. Induction of apoptosis by *D*-limonene is mediated by inactivation of Akt in LS174T human colon cancer cells. Oncology Reports. 2013;**3**(23):349-354

[22] Yang C, Chen H, Chen H, Zhong B, Luo X, Chun J. Antioxidant and anticancer activities of essential oil from gannan navel orange peel. Molecules. 2017;**22**(8):1-10. DOI: 10.3310.3390/molecules22081391

[23] Miller JA, Pappan K, Thompson PA, Want EJ, Siskos AP, Keun HC, et al. Plasma metabolomic pro files of breast cancer patients after short-term limonene intervention. Cancer Prevention Research (Philadelphia, Pa.). 2015;**8**(1):86-93. DOI: 10.1158/1940-6207

[24] Haag JD, Lindstrom MJ, Gould MN, Haag JD, Lindstrom MJ, Gould MN. Limonene-induced regression of mammary carcinomas limonene-induced regression of mammary carcinomas. Cancer Research. 1992;**52**(14):4021-4026

[25] Gould N, Moore J, Kennan S, Haag JD. Limonene chemoprevention of mammary carcinoma induction following direct in situ transfer of v-ha-ras1. Cancer Research. 1994;**54**(13):3540-3543

[26] Yuri T, Danbara N, Tsujita-kyutoku M, Kiyozuka Y, Shikata N, Kanzaki H, et al. Perillyl alcohol inhibits human breast cancer cell growth *in vitro* and *in vivo*. Breast Cancer Research and Treatment. 2004;**84**(3):251-260

[27] Thomadaki H, Talieri M, Scorilas A. Treatment of MCF-7 cells with taxol and etoposide induces distinct alterations in the expression of apoptosis-related genes BCL2, BCL2L12, BAX, CASPASE-9 and FAS. Biological Chemistry. 2006;**387**(8):1081-1086. DOI: 10.1515/BC.2006.133

[28] Tudor G, Aguilera A, Halverson DO, Laing ND. Susceptibility to drug-induced apoptosis correlates with differential modulation of Bad, Bcl-2 and Bcl-x L protein levels. Cell Death and Differentiation. 2000;**7**(6):574-586. DOI: 10.1038/sj.cdd.4400688

[29] Ofir R, Seidman R, Rabinski T, Krup M, Yavelsky V, Weinstein Y, et al. Taxol-induced apoptosis in human SKOV3 ovarian and MCF7 breast carcinoma cells is caspase-3 and

caspase-9 independent. Cell Death and Differentiation. 2002;**9**:636-642

[30] Flores ML, Castilla C, Ávila R, Ruiz-Borrego M, Sáez C, Japón MA. Paclitaxel sensitivity of breast cancer cells requires efficient mitotic arrest and disruption of Bcl-xL/Bak interaction. Breast Cancer Research and Treatment. 2012;**133**(3):917-928. DOI: 10.1007/s10549-011-1864-9

[31] Barbuti AM, Chen Z. Paclitaxel through the ages of anticancer therapy: Exploring its role in chemoresistance and radiation therapy. Cancers (Basel). 2015;7(4):2360-2371. DOI: 10.3390/cancers7040897

[32] Weaver B. How taxol/paclitaxel kills cancer cells. Molecular Biology of the Cell. 2014;**25**(18):2677-2681. DOI: 10.1091/mbc.E14-04-0916

[33] Luo J, Hu YANL, Wang H. Ursolic acid inhibits breast cancer growth by inhibiting proliferation, inducing autophagy and apoptosis, and suppressing inflammatory responses via the PI3K/AKT and NF-κ B signaling pathways *in vitro*. Experimental and Therapeutic Medicine. 2017;**14**: 3623-3631. DOI: 10.3892/etm.2017.4965

[34] Pironi AM, Araújo PR De, Fernandes MA. Nunes Salgado RA and Chorilli M. Characteristics, biological properties and analytical methods of ursolic acid: A review. Critical Reviews in Analytical Chemistry. 2017:1-25. DOI: 10.1080/10408347.2017.1390425

[35] Hasanpourghadi M, Kumar A, Rais M. Modulation of oncogenic transcription factors by bioactive natural products in breast cancer. Pharmacological Research. 2018; **128, 128**:376-388. DOI: 10.1016/j.phrs.2017.09.009

[36] Lewinska A, Adamczyk J, Ewa G. Ursolic acid-mediated changes in glycolytic pathway promote cytotoxic autophagy and apoptosis in phenotypically different breast cancer cells. Apoptosis. 2017. DOI: 10.1007/s10495-017-1353-7

[37] Subramani R, Lakshmanaswamy R. Complementary and alternative medicine and breast cancer. Progress in Molecular Biology and Translational Science. 2017:1-44. DOI: 10.1016/bs.pmbts.2017.07.008

[38] Surh Y-J. Cancer chemoprevention with dietary phytochemicals. Nature Reviews. 2003;**3**:768-780. DOI: 10.1038/nrc1189

[39] Forcados GE, James DB, Sallau AB, Muhammad A, Mabeta P. Oxidative stress and carcinogenesis: Potential of phytochemicals in breast cancer therapy. Nutrition and Cancer. 2017:1-10. DOI: 10.1080/01635581.2017.1267777

[40] Assar EA, Vidalle MC, Chopra M, Hafizi S. Lycopene acts through inhibition of IκB kinase to suppress NF-κ B signaling in human prostate and breast cancer cells. Tumor Biology. 2016;**37**(7):9375-9385. DOI: 10.1007/s13277-016-4798-3

[41] Estanislao Gómez CC, Aquino Carreño A, Pérez Ishiwara DG, San Martín Martínez E, Morales López J, Pérez Hernández N, et al. Decatropis bicolor (Zucc) radlk essential oil induces apoptosis of the MDA-MB-231 breast cancer cell line. BMC Complementary and Alternative Medicine. 2016;**16**(1):266-276. DOI: 10.1186/s12906-016-1136-7

[42] Goodarzi S, Tabatabaei MJ, Jafari RM, Shemirani F, Tavakoli S, Mofasseri M, et al. Cuminum cyminum fruits as source of luteolin-7-O-glucoside, potent cytotoxic flavonoid against breast cancer cell lines. Natural Product Research. 2018:1-5. DOI: 10.1080/14786419.2018.1519824

[43] Wang RUI, Wang J, Dong T, Shen JUN, Gao X, Zhou JUN. Naringenin has a chemoprotective effect in MDA-MB-231 breast cancer cells via inhibition of caspase-3 and -9 activities. Oncology Letters. 2019;**17**:1217-1222. DOI: 10.3892/ol.2018.9704

[44] Ren G, Shi Z, Cong T, Yao Y. Antiproliferative activity of combined Biochanin A and Ginsenoside Rh2 on MDA-MB-231 and MCF-7 human breast cancer cells. Molecules. 2018;**23**(2908):1-14. DOI: 10.3390/molecules23112908

[45] Chen J, Ge B, Wang Y, Ye Y, Zeng S, Huang Z. Biochanin a promotes proliferation that involves a feedback loop of MicroRNA-375 and estrogen receptor alpha in breast cancer cells. Cellular Physiology and Biochemistry. 2015;**35**:639-646. DOI: 10.1159/000369725

[46] Pfeffer CM, Singh ATK. Apoptosis: A target for anticancer therapy. International Journal of Molecular Sciences. 2018;**19**:1-10. DOI: 10.3390/ijms19020448 2018;2

[47] Fang Y, Zhang Q, Wang X, Yang X, Wang X, Huang Z, et al. Quantitative phosphoproteomics reveals genistein as a modulator of cell cycle and DNA damage response pathways in triple-negative breast cancer cells. International Journal of Oncology. 2016;**48**:1016-1028. DOI: 10.3892/ijo.2016.3327

[48] Jiang H, Fan J, Cheng L. The anticancer activity of genistein is increased in estrogen receptor beta 1-positive breast cancer cells. OncoTargets and Therapy. 2018;**11**:8153-8163

[49] Jain A, Sharma G, Ghoshal G, Kesharwani P, Singh B, Shivhare US, et al. Lycopene loaded whey protein isolate nanoparticles: An innovative endeavor for enhanced bioavailability of lycopene and anti-cancer activity. International Journal of Pharmaceutics. 2018;**30**(546):97-105. DOI: 10.1016/j.ijpharm

[50] Sheihet L, Garbuzenko OB, Bushman J, Gounder MK, Minko T, Kohn J. European journal of pharmaceutical sciences paclitaxel in tyrosine-derived nanospheres as a potential anti-cancer agent: *In vivo* evaluation of toxicity and efficacy in comparison with paclitaxel in cremophor. European Journal of Pharmaceutical Sciences. 2012;**45**(3):320-329. DOI: 10.1016/j.ejps.2011.11.017

[51] Pozo-Guisado E, Centeno F, Merino JM, Mulero-navarro S, Jesu M, Alvarez-barrientos A, et al. Resveratrol-induced apoptosis in MCF-7 human breast cancer cells involves a caspase-independent mechanism with downregulation of Bcl-2 and NF-kB. International Journal of Cancer. 2005;**115**(1):74-84

[52] Jones CB, Clements MK, Wasi S, Daoud SS. Enhancement of camptothecin-induced cytotoxicity with UCN-01 in breast cancer cells: Abrogation of S/G2 arrest. Cancer Chemotherapy and Pharmacology. 2000;**45**(3):252-258

[53] Chu C, Xu J, Cheng D, Li X, Tong S, Yan J, et al. Anti-proliferative and apoptosis-inducing effects of camptothecin-20(s)-*O*-(2-pyrazolyl-1) acetic ester in human breast tumor MCF-7 cells. Molecules. 2014;**19**(4):4941-4955. DOI: 10.3390/molecules19044941

[54] Ramachandran C, Rodriguez S, Ramachandran R, Nair PKR, Fonseca H, Khatib Z, et al. Expression profiles of apoptotic genes induced by curcumin in human breast cancer and mammary epithelial cell lines. Anticancer Research. 2005;**25**(5):3293-3302

[55] Prasad CP, Rath G, Mathur S, Bhatnagar D, Ralhan R. Chemico-biological interactions potent growth suppressive activity of curcumin in human breast cancer cells: Modulation of Wnt/beta-catenin signaling. Chemico-Biological Interactions. 2009;**181**(2):263-271. DOI: 10.1016/j.cbi.2009.06.012

[56] Groth-Pedersen L, Ostenfeld MS, Høyer-Hansen M, Nylandsted J, Jäättelä M. Vincristine induces dramatic lysosomal changes and sensitizes cancer cells to lysosome-destabilizing siramesine. Cancer Research. 2007;**67**(5):2217-2225

[57] Lin H-Y, Lansing L, Merillon J-M, Davis FB, Tang H-Y, Shih A, et al. Integrin αVβ3 contains a receptor site for resveratrol. The FASEB Journal. 2006;**20**(10):1742-1744. DOI: 10.1096/fj.06-5743fje

[58] Dong Z. Molecular mechanism of the chemopreventive effect of resveratrol. Mutation Research. 2003;**524**:145-150

[59] Gambini J, Inglés M, Olaso G, Abdelaziz KM, Vina J, Borras C. Properties of resveratrol: *In vitro* and *in vivo* studies about metabolism, bioavailability, and biological effects in animal models and humans. Oxidative Medicine and Cellular Longevity. 2015;**2015**:837042. DOI: 10.1155/2015/837042

[60] Nakagawa H, Kiyozuka Y, Uemura Y, Senzaki H, Shikata N, Hioki K, et al. Resveratrol inhibits human breast cancer cell growth and may mitigate the effect of linoleic acid, a potent breast cancer cell stimulator. Journal of Cancer Research and Clinical Oncology. 2001;**127**(4):258-264

[61] Alkhalaf M. Resveratrol-induced growth inhibition in MDA-MB-231 breast cancer cells is associated with mitogen-activated protein kinase signaling and protein translation. European Journal of Cancer Prevention. 2007;**16**(4):334-341

[62] Garvin S, Ollinger K, Dabrosin C. Resveratrol induces apoptosis and inhibits angiogenesis in human breast cancer xenografts *in vivo*. Cancer Letters. 2006;**231**(1):113-122. DOI: 10.1016/j.canlet.2005.01.031

[63] Cal C, Garban H, Jazirehi A, Yeh C, Mizutani Y, Bonavida B. Resveratrol and cancer: Chemoprevention, apoptosis, and chemo-immunosensitizing activities. Current Medicinal Chemistry. Anti-Cancer Agents. 2003;**3**(2):77-93

[64] Ko J-H, Sethi G, Um J-Y, Shanmugam MK, Arfuso F, Alan Prem Kumar AB, et al. The role of resveratrol in cancer therapy. International Journal of Molecular Sciences. 2017;**18**(2589):1-36. DOI: 10.3390/ijms18122589

[65] Bhat KP, Lantvit D, Christov K, Mehta RG, Moon RC, Pezzuto JM. Estrogenic and antiestrogenic properties of resveratrol in mammary tumor models. Cancer Research. 2001;**61**(20):7456-7463

[66] Provinciali M, Re F, Donnini A, Orlando F, Bartozzi B, Di Stasio G, et al. Effect of resveratrol on the development of spontaneous mammary tumors in HER-2/neutransgenic mice. International Journal of Cancer. 2005;**115**(1):36-45. DOI: 10.1002/ijc.20874

[67] Banerjee S, Bueso-Ramos C, Aggarwal BB. Carcinogenesis in rats by resveratrol role of nuclear factor-kappa B, suppression of 7,12-dimethylbenz(a)anthracene-induced mammary carcinogenesis in rats by resveratrol: Role of nuclear factor-kappa B, cyclooxygenase 2, and matrix metalloprotease 9. International Journal of Cancer. 2002;**62**(17):4945-4954

[68] Chatterjee M, Chatterjee M, Das S, Janarthan M, Ramachandran HK. Role of 5-lipoxygenase in resveratrol mediated suppression of 7,12-dimethylbenz(α)anthracene-induced mammary carcinogenesis in rats. European Journal of Pharmacology. 2011;**668**:99-106. DOI: 10.1016/j.ejphar.2011.06.039

[69] Nguyen AV, Martinez M, Stamos MJ, Moyer MP, Hope C, Holcombe RF. Results of a phase I pilot clinical trial examining the effect of plant-derived resveratrol and grape powder on Wnt pathway target gene expression in colonic mucosa and colon cancer. Cancer Management and Research. 2009;**3**(1):25-37

[70] Berman AY, Motechin RA, Wiesenfeld MY, Holz MK. The therapeutic potential of resveratrol: A review of clinical trials. NPJ Precision Oncology. 2017;**1**:1-9. DOI: 10.1038/s41698-017-0038-6

[71] Shanmugam MK, Rane G, Kanchi MM, Arfuso F, Chinnathambi A, Zayed ME, et al. The multifaceted role of Curcumin in cancer prevention and treatment. Molecules. 2015;**20**(2):2728-2769. DOI: 10.3390/molecules20022728

[72] Liu H, Ho Y. Food science and human wellness anticancer effect of curcumin on breast cancer and stem cells. Food Science and Human Wellness. 2018;**7**(2):134-137. DOI: 10.1016/j.fshw.2018.06.001

[73] Ravindran J, Prasad S, Aggarwal BB. Curcumin and cancer cells: How many ways can curry kill tumor cells selectively? The AAPS Journal. 2009;**11**(3):495-510. DOI: 10.1208/s12248-009-9128-x

[74] Karunagaran D, Rashmi R, Kumar T. Induction of apoptosis by curcumin and its implications for cancer therapy. Current Cancer Drug Targets. 2005;**5**(2):117-129

[75] Khan MA, Gahlot S, Majumdar S. Oxidative stress induced by curcumin promotes the death of cutaneous T-cell lymphoma (HuT-78) by disrupting the function of several molecular targets. Molecular Cancer Therapeutics. 2012;**11**(9):1873-1883. DOI: 10.1158/1535-7163

[76] Chakraborty G, Jain S, Kale S, Raja R, Kumar S, Mishra R, et al. Curcumin suppresses breast tumor angiogenesis by abrogating osteopontin-induced VEGF expression. Molecular Medicine Reports. 2008;**1**(5):641-646. DOI: 10.3892/mmr_00000005

[77] Kunnumakkara AB, Anand P, Aggarwal BB. Curcumin inhibits proliferation, invasion, angiogenesis and metastasis of different cancers through interaction with multiple cell signaling proteins. Cancer Letters. 2008;**269**(2):199-225. DOI: 10.1016/j.canlet.2008.03.009

[78] Hua W, Fu Y, Liao Y, Xia W, Chen Y, Zeng Y, et al. Curcumin induces down-regulation of EZH2 expression through the MAPK pathway in MDA-MB-435 human breast cancer cells. European Journal of Pharmacology. 2010;**637**(1-3):16-21. DOI: 10.1016/j.ejphar.2010.03.05179

[79] Banerjee M, Singh P, Panda D. Curcumin suppresses the dynamic instability of microtubules, activates the mitotic checkpoint and induces apoptosis in MCF-7 cells. The FEBS Journal. 2010;**277**(16):3437-3448. DOI: 10.1111/j.1742-4658.2010.07750

[80] Habli Z, Toumieh G, Fatfat M, Rahal ON, Gali-Muhtasib H. Emerging cytotoxic alkaloids in the battle against cancer: Overview of molecular mechanisms. Molecules. 2017;**22**(2):1-22. DOI: 10.3390/molecules22020250

[81] Wink M. Modes of action of herbal medicines and plant secondary metabolites. Medicine. 2015;**2**(3):

[82] Aniszewski T. Alkaloids. Secrets of Life. Alkaloid Chemistry, Biological Significance, Applications and Ecological Role. Amsterdam: Elsevier; 2007. p. 316

[83] Mohan K, Jeyachandran R. Alkaloids as anticancer agents. Annals of Phytomedicine. 2012;**1**(1):46-53

[84] Legarza K, Yang L. New molecular mechanisms of action of camptothecin-type drugs. Anticancer Research. 2006;**26**(5A):3301-3305

[85] Sirikantaramas S, Yamazaki M, Saito K. Mutations in topoisomerase I as a self-resistance mechanism coevolved with the production of the anticancer alkaloid camptothecin in plants. Proceedings of the National Academy of Sciences of the United States of America. 2008;**105**(18):6782-6786. DOI: 10.1073/pnas.0801038105

[86] Liu LF, Desai SD, Li TK, Mao Y, Sun M, Sim S. Mechanism of action of camptothecin. Annals of the New York Academy of Sciences. 2000;**922**:1-10

[87] Burke TG, Xiang TX, Anderson BD, Latus LJ. Recent advances in camptothecin drug design and delivery strategies. camptothecins in cancer therapy. Human Press. 2005:171-190. DOI: 10.1385/1-59259-866-8:171

[88] Giovanella BC, Hinz HR, Kozielski AJ, Stehlin JS, Silber R, Potmesil M. Complete growth inhibition of human cancer inhibition of human cancer xenografts in nude mice by treatment with 20-(5-camptothecin). Cancer Research. 1991;**5**:3052-3056

[89] Venditto VJ, Simanek EE. Cancer therapies utilizing the camptothecins: A review of *in vivo* literature. Molecular Pharmaceutics. 2010;7(2):307-349. DOI: 10.1021/mp900243b

251-286. DOI: 10.3390/medicines2030251

[90] Lee C, Huang Y, Yang C, Huang K. Drug delivery systems and combination therapy by using vinca alkaloids. Current Topics in Medicinal Chemistry. 2015;**15**(15):1491-1500. DOI: 10.2174/1568026615666150414120547

[91] Moudi M, Go R, Yien CY, Nazre M. Vinca alkaloids. International Journal of Preventive Medicine. 2013;**4**(11):1231-1235

[92] Downing KH. Structural basis for the interaction of tubulin with proteins and drugs that affect microtubule dynamics. Annual Review of Cell and Developmental Biology. 2000;**16**:89-111

[93] Gregory RK, Smith IE. Vinorelbina: A clinical review. British Journal of Cancer. 2000;**82**:1907-1913

[94] Klement G, Baruchel S, Rak J, Man S, Clark K, Hicklin DJ, et al. Erratum: Continuous low-dose therapy with vinblastine and VEGF receptor-2 antibody induces sustained tumor regression without overt toxicity. The Journal of Clinical Investigation. 2000;**105**:R15-R24. DOI: 10.1172/JCI08829C1

[95] Sen K, Mandal M. Second generation liposomal cancer therapeutics: Transition from laboratory to clinic. International Journal of Pharmaceutics. 2013;**448**(1):28-43. DOI: 10.1016/j.ijpharm.2013.03.006

[96] Allen TM, Cullis PR. Liposomal drug delivery systems: From concept to clinical applications. Advanced Drug Delivery Reviews. 2013;**65**(1):36-48. DOI: 10.1016/j.addr.2012.09.037

[97] Shaban N, Abdel-Rahman S, Haggag A, Awad D, Bassiouny A, Talaat I. Combination between Taxol-encapsulated liposomes and Eruca sativa seed extract suppresses mammary tumors in female rats induced by 7,12-dimethylbenz(α)anthracene. Asian Pacific Journal of

Cancer Prevention. 2016;**17**(1): 117-123

[98] Singh B, Shoulson R, Chatterjee A, Ronghe A, Bhat NK, Dim DC, et al. Resveratrol inhibits estrogen-induced breast carcinogenesis through induction of NRF2-mediated protective pathways. Carcinogenesis. 2014;**35**(8):1872-1880. DOI: 10.1093/carcin/bgu120

[99] Zhou QM, Wang XF, Liu XJ, Zhang H, Lu YY, Su SB. Curcumin enhanced antiproliferative effect of mitomycin C in human breast cancer MCF-7 cells *in vitro* and *in vivo*. Acta Pharmacologica Sinica. 2011;**32**(11):1402-1410. DOI: 10.1038/aps.2011.97

[100] Camacho KM, Kumar S, Menegatti S, Vogus DG, Anselmo AC, Mitragotri S. Synergistic Antitumor Activity of Camptothecin-Doxorubicin Combinations and their Conjugates with Hyaluronic Acid. Journal of Controlled Release. 2015:1-25. DOI:10.1016/j.jconrel.2015.04.031

[101] Ping M, Russell M. Paclitaxel Nano-delivery systems: A comprehensive review. Journal of Nanomedicine & Nanotechnology. 2013;**4**(2):1000164. DOI: 10.4172/2157-7439.1000164

[102] Sofias AM, Dunne M, Storm G, Allen G. The battle of "nano" paclitaxel. Advanced Drug Delivery Reviews. 2017;**122**:20-30. DOI: 10.1016/j.addr.2017.02.003

[103] Wu C, Gao Y, Liu Y, Xu X. Pure paclitaxel nanoparticles: Preparation, characterization, and antitumor effect for human liver cancer SMMC-7721 cells. International Journal of Nanomedicine. 2018;**13**:6189-6198. DOI: 10.2147/IJN.S169209

[104] Wang F, Porter M, Konstantopoulos A, Zhang P, Cui H. Preclinical development of drug delivery systems for paclitaxel-based cancer chemotherapy. Journal of Controlled Release. 2017;**267**:100-118. DOI: 10.1016/j.jconrel.2017.09.026

[105] Shen J, Sun H, Xu P, Yin Q, Zhang Z, Wang S, et al. Biomaterials simultaneous inhibition of metastasis and growth of breast cancer by co-delivery of twist shRNA and paclitaxel using pluronic P85-PEI/TPGS complex nanoparticles. Biomaterials. 2012;**34**(5):1581-1590. DOI: 10.1016/j.biomaterials.2012.10.057

[106] Mahalingam M, Krishnamoorthy K. Selection of a suitable method for the preparation of polymeric nanoparticles: Multi-criteria decision making approach. Advanced Pharmaceutical Bulletin. 2015;**5**(1):57-67. DOI: 10.5681/apb.2015.008

[107] Acevedo-Morantes CY, Acevedo-Morantes MT, Suleiman-Rosado D, Ramírez-Vick JE. Evaluation of the cytotoxic effect of camptothecin solid lipid nanoparticles on MCF7 cells. Drug Delivery. 2013;**20**(8):338-348. DOI: 10.3109/10717544.2013.834412

[108] Mohanty C, Sahoo SK. The *in vitro* stability and *in vivo* pharmacokinetics of curcumin prepared as an aqueous nanoparticulate formulation. Biomaterials. 2010;**31**(25):6597-6611. DOI: 10.1016/j.biomaterials.2010.04.062

[109] Manikandan M, Kannan K. Pharmacokinetic and pharmacodynamic evaluation of camptothecin encapsulated poly (methacylic acid-co-methyl methacrylate) nanoparticles. Journal of Applied Pharmaceutical Science. 2017;**7**(3):9-16. DOI: 10.7324/JAPS.2017.70303

[110] Mulik RS, Mönkkönen J, Juvonen RO, Mahadik KR, Paradkar AR. Transferrin mediated solid lipid nanoparticles containing curcumin: Enhanced *in vitro* anticancer

activity by induction of apoptosis. International Journal of Pharmaceutics. 2010;**398**(1-2):190-203. DOI: 10.1016/j.ijpharm.2010.07.021

[111] Tang H, Murphy CJ, Zhang B, Shen Y, Van Kirk EA, Murdoch WJ, et al. Biomaterials Curcumin polymers as anticancer conjugates. Biomaterials. 2010;**31**(27):7139-7149. DOI: 10.1016/j.biomaterials.2010.06.007

[112] Ducry L, Stump B. Antibody—Drug conjugates: Linking cytotoxic payloads to monoclonal antibodies. Bioconjugate Chemistry. 2010;**21**:5-13. DOI: 10.1021/bc9002019

Chapter 5

Apoptotic Inhibitors as Therapeutic Targets for Cell Survival

El-Shimaa Mohamed Naguib Abdelhafez,
Sara Mohamed Naguib Abdelhafez Ali,
Mohamed Ramadan Eisa Hassan and
Adel Mohammed Abdel-Hakem

Abstract

Apoptosis has revealed an essential function in the development or prevention of oncogenic transformation in the body; however, programmed cell death (PCD) must be tightly controlled since deregulated cell death is involved in the development of a large number of different pathologies. Apoptosis can be decreased in pathological states such as in cancer and autoimmunity or elevated such as in stroke, neurodegeneration, retinal cell death, myocardial and liver ischemia, inflammatory diseases such as sepsis, osteoarthritis (OA), rheumatoid arthritis (RA), and asthma. Different types of apoptotic inhibitors will be discussed in this chapter displaying their mechanism of action, which have been reported to be therapeutic targets for cell survival or at least limiting cell death. These inhibitors are classified according to their nature into natural antiapoptotic proteins that present mainly in the cell and synthetic small molecule inhibitors that are widely used to protect against overexpression of apoptosis mediators and, in turn, to prevent corresponding diseases.

Keywords: antiapoptosis, mechanism, apoptotic inhibitors, endogenous, synthetic, cell survival

1. Introduction

Apoptosis is a crucial normal biological process that occurs in the cell as a component of animal development, tissue hemostasis, and immune response. In pathological state, it can be abrogated as in cancer and autoimmune diseases, or over-expressed as in case of stroke, ischemia, psoriasis, and inflammatory diseases.

The apoptotic mechanism occurs through either extrinsic pathway or intrinsic pathway, which leads to cell death through different apoptotic cascades, according to the type of stimuli [1].

These cell survival strategies involve a myriad of coordinated and systematic physiological and genetic changes that serve to ward off death [2].

There are various inhibitors of these pathways, which have been reported to be helpful in inhibition of the cell death or limiting it. These inhibitors are classified according to their nature into endogenous antiapoptotic proteins that present mainly in the cell to regulate the apoptosis process and synthetic inhibitors that are synthesized to be used in case of overexpression of apoptosis mediators as in some diseases.

1.1 Endogenous antiapoptotic inhibitors

1.1.1 Reduction in the number of apoptotic cells

It was reported that *Ginkgo biloba* extract (EGb 761) exhibited antiapoptotic effect on different cell types [3], and it particularly inhibits death in human lymphocytes when exposed to gossypol, a toxin that causes cell death via apoptosis. Similar results have been observed in thymus cells pretreated with EGb 761 and then exposed to ferrous sulfate in hydrogen peroxide (H_2O_2) [4]. Lymphocytes that are isolated from spleen of aged mice and treated with EGb 761 were less susceptible to reactive oxygen species (ROS)-induced apoptosis [5]. Scientists revealed that the posttreatment with EGb 761 in the peripheral nervous system decreased efficiently the number of apoptotic cells in injured rat spinal cord [6]. Moreover, it helps in treatment of the central nervous system reduced neuronal death in the *substantia nigra pars compacta* from an experimental model of Parkinson's disease [7].

1.1.2 Maintaining the mitochondrial integrity

Rhodiola crenulata extract (RCE) is an edible alcohol extract, conserving greatly the mitochondrial integrity and in turn prohibiting the release of cytochrome C, which leads to cell death. The effective concentration of the most important component, salidroside, was ~4% (w/w).

Other herbals mediate its antiapoptotic effect through the same mechanism as they possess a potent reactive oxygen species scavenging function; however, they restore the mitochondrial membrane potential [8, 9].

Some drugs were tested in sympathoadrenal cells that showed obviously another antiapoptotic pathway through inducing the antiapoptotic protein B-cell lymphoma 2 (Bcl-2) transcription rate and B-cell lymphoma-extra-large (Bcl-xL) proteins. The role of these proteins appears crucial, because inhibition of their production by antisense oligonucleotides (directed toward the translation initiation site of the Bcl-2 transcript) resulted in abolishing protective effect. The prosurvival pathway also included activation of the transcription nuclear factors NF-κB (a protein complex that controls transcription of DNA, cytokine production, and cell survival) and CREB (cellular transcription factor). It binds to certain DNA sequences and the antiapoptotic kinase PKCα/β such as dehydroepiandrosterone (DHEAS) and Allo [10].

1.1.3 Decrease in caspase transcription rate and DNA fragmentation

Some natural component reverse such as diosmin induces Bad and Bax, proapoptotic members of the Bcl-2 family, to react with the mitochondrial membrane and prevent the release of apoptotic-inducing factor (AIF) and cytochrome-C. Cytochrome-C in turn inhibits initiator caspase-9, which prevents sequential cascade of activation of caspase-3, and conserves DNA fragment along with no apoptotic cell death [11].

1.2 Synthetic apoptotic inhibitors

1.2.1 Tumor necrotic factor (TNF) inhibitors

Infliximab (IFX) [12], etanercept (ETN) [13], Adalimumab (ADA), golimumab (GOLI) [14], and certolizumab pegol (CZP) [15] are clinical biologic drugs that act as necrotic factor (TNF)-α inhibitors that were approved by the U.S. Food and Drug Administration (FDA). Other synthetic TNF inhibitors were designed such as:

Compound (1) inhibited the release of TNF in cells and in animals. It was active in a chronic rheumatoid arthritis model (MCIA) when administrated orally and it was advanced for further preclinical evaluation [16]. A novel thalidomide analog was synthesized and characterized for anti-TNF-α activity with up to a 38% inhibition for compound (2) with no obvious concentration dependence [17].

Compound (3) is an oleanolic acid analog, characterized by structural modifications at position C-3 and C-28 of oleanane skeleton and tested for anti-inflammatory potential, when C-3 became Indole, and C-28 = cyclohexamine, gave mild inhibition by 51.9% [18]. Compound (4) suppressed serum TNF-α levels by 2.45 ng/ml compared to the control group 5.61 ng/ml [19].

Compound (5) possessed TNF inhibition with half-maximal inhibitory concentration (IC50) = 0.5 μm [19]. Besides, Compound (6) decreased the level of the pro-inflammatory cytokine TNF-α by (39.19%) [20].

Compound (7) had 56% inhibition of TNF-α at 10 μm [21]. Betulinic acid (8) had a significant decrease in IL1β, IL6, and TNFα in the neuronal tissues [22].

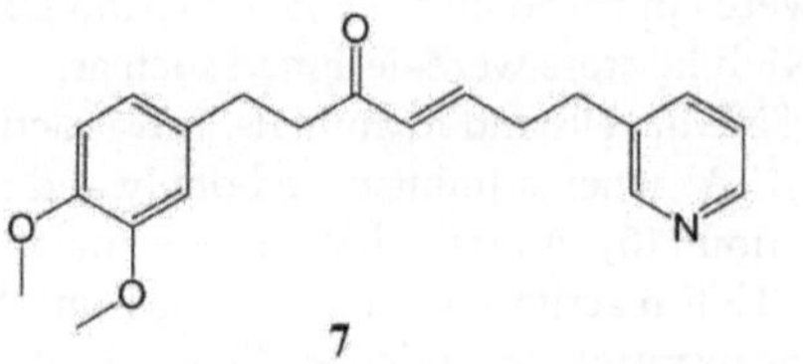

7

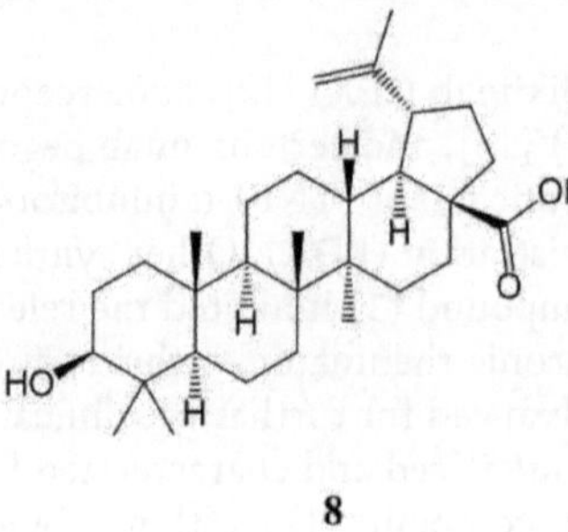

8

1.2.2 Fatty acid synthase (Fas) inhibitors

KR-33493 (9) was used as a potent inhibitor for ischemia Fas-mediated cell death 68 [23]. Compound (10a, b) RKTS-33,34 with 10 μm ED50 value (concentration causing 50% of maximum effect) selectively inhibited apoptosis induced by FasL as well as ECH (epoxycyclohexenone derivative) (11), which is produced by fungus [24].

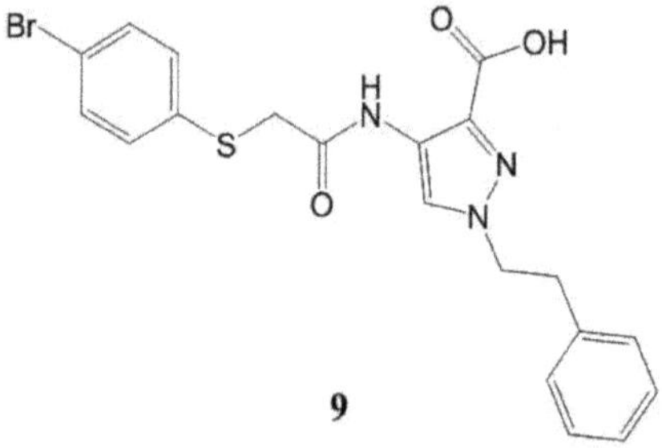

9

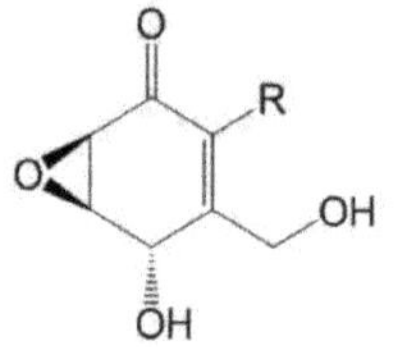

a= RKTS-33 R = H
b= RKTS-34 R = -C(CH3)=CH-CH3

10

Glycine (12) was tested as a cytoprotector against ischemic damage by downregulation of FasL/Fas and caspase3 and upregulation of Bcl2 and Bcl2-bax (apoptosis regulator BAX) [25]. Compound (13) was designed as a novel class of ischemic cell death inhibitors targeting Fas-mediated cell death pathway with EC50 = 0.557 μm (the concentration of a drug that gives half-maximal response), and cell survival = 92.98% at 10 μm [26]. It was found that (dichlorovinyl dimethyl phosphate) DDVP (14) significantly decreased the expression of Fas antigen on YAC-1S target cells and the expression of FasL (Fas ligand) on LAK cells (lymphokine-activated killer cell). These findings provided direct evidences that DDVP impaired the FasL/Fas pathway via downregulating the expression of both Fas and FasL [27]. Geldanamycin (15), which was originally discovered in Streptomyces hygroscopicus [28], inhibited Fas signaling pathway and protected neurons against ischemia [29].

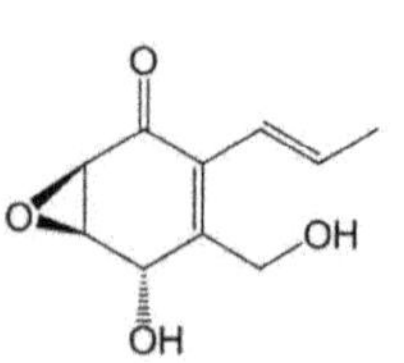

11

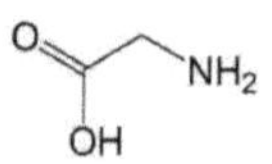

12

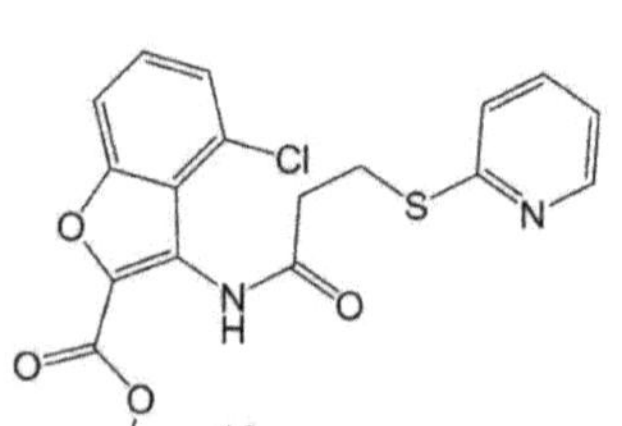

13

DDVP
14

Geldanamycin
15

Compound (16) is the active form of vitamin D that inhibited Fas ligand-induced apoptosis in human osteoblasts by regulating components of both the mitochondrial and Fas-related pathways [30]. Estrogen (17) also inhibited Fas-mediated apoptosis in experimental stroke [31].

16

VIt. D3 (active form)

Estrogen
17

Cilazapril (18) acts as an angiotensin-converting enzyme inhibitor along with protection against apoptosis through downregulating Fas protein during the induction of apoptosis in cardiomyocytes in rat hearts when subjected to reperfusion after ischemia [32]. M50054 (19) (cell-permeable inhibitor of the activation of caspase-3) inhibited apoptosis induced by a variety of apoptotic stimuli such as the Fas/Fas ligand system and etoposide. Thus, it might be effective for hepatitis when administered orally and chemotherapy-induced alopecia when administered topically [33].

Cilazapril
18

M50054
19

SC79 (20) (AKT activator) prevented acute hepatic failure induced by Fas-mediated apoptosis of hepatocytes [34]. Vit K2 (21) significantly suppressed both Fas expression and Fas-mediated apoptosis of the cells in a dose-dependent fashion. The maximum effect was observed when 6–10 mol/L of vitamin K2 was added to the culture, a concentration comparable to that attained during therapy with vitamin K2 [35].

Vanillic acid (22) inhibited Fas-receptor and caspase-mediated apoptosis signaling pathway and so acted as cardioprotective [36]. NCX-1000 (NO-releasing derivative of ursodeoxycholic acid) (23) is a nitric oxide (NO) derivative of ursodeoxycholic acid (UDCA). When an NO-releasing moiety is added to UDCA, the effectiveness in preventing Fas-mediated liver injury increased [37].

1.2.3 BH3 interacting-domain death agonist (BID) inhibitors

BID plays a central role in the apoptotic machinery mediating cytochrome C and SMAC/DIABLO (mitochondrial protein that potentiates some forms of apoptosis) released from mitochondria, a crucial event for caspase activation and cell death [38]. Pharmacological inhibition of BID could therefore provide a protective benefit against pathological cell death, occurring in cerebral ischemia [39], neurodegenerative diseases [40, 41], liver inflammation [42], or other illnesses where BID has been implicated [43].

BI-6C9 (24) was effective in inhibiting the carboxyl-terminal fragment (tBid) (truncated protein) association with isolated mitochondria at 20 μm [39]. TC9-305 (2-sulfonyl-pyrimidinyl derivatives) (25) had an EC50 = 0.23 nm [44]. BI-11A7 (26) was much more effective in this assay when compared with BI-6C9 (24) but showed some toxicity at higher concentrations (20 μm) [45]. 3-o-tolylthiazolidine-

2,4-dione (27) protected neural cells against glutamate- and tBid-induced toxicity with an EC50 = 6.78 μm [46].

BI-6C9

24

25

TC9-305

27

26

BI-11A7

1.2.4 Tumor necrosis factor-like weak inducer of apoptosis (TWEAK) inhibitors

TWEAK also known as (Apo3L or TNFSF12) was first described as an inducer of apoptosis in transformed cell lines [47]. It is a member of the tumor necrosis factor (TNF) receptor family that is induced in a variety of cell types in situations of tissue injury. It is a crucial player in muscle atrophy, cerebral ischemia, kidney injury, atherosclerosis, and infarction, as well as in various autoimmune scenarios including experimental autoimmune encephalitis, rheumatoid arthritis, and inflammatory bowel disease [48]. Aurintricarboxylic acid (ATA) (28) was a potent inhibitor of the TWEAK-Fn14 signaling axis and could potentially be utilized to enhance the therapeutic response in glioblastoma (GBM) [49]. L524-0366 (29) was a specific dose-dependent inhibitor of TWEAK-Fn14 interaction [50] and it was found to be a complete suppressor for TWEAK-induced T98G cell migration at dose equal to 10 μm [51].

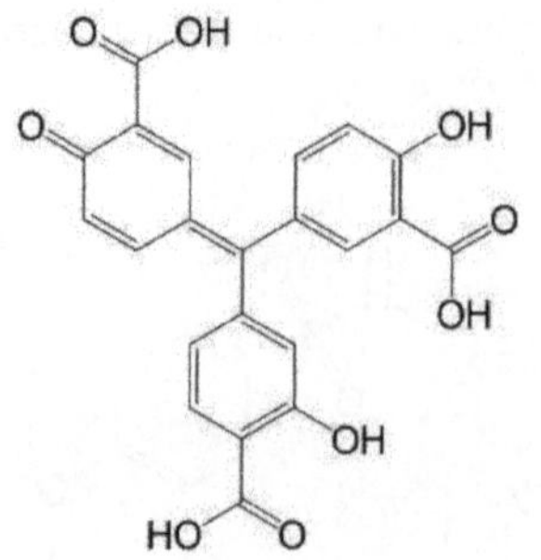

ATA 28

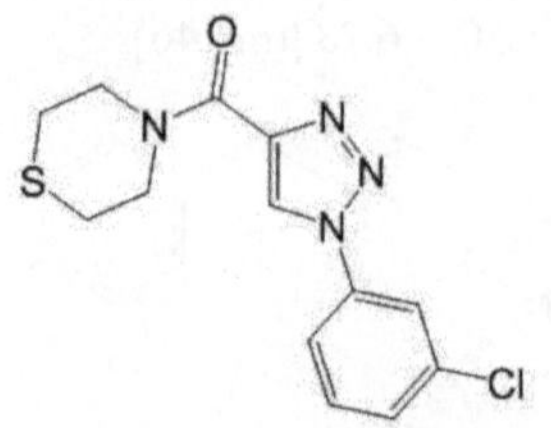

L524-0366 29

1.2.5 Cytochrome C inhibitors

Cytochrome C is the specific and efficient electron transfer mediator between the two last redox complexes of the mitochondrial respiratory chain [52]. The release of cytochrome C from the mitochondria into the cytoplasm results in caspase-9 activation leading to cell death [43]. Minocycline (30) directly inhibited the release of cytochrome C from mitochondria. Therefore, it was beneficial in experimental models of stroke, traumatic brain and spinal cord injury, Huntington's disease (HD), amyotrophic lateral sclerosis (ALS), Parkinson's disease, and multiple sclerosis [53, 54]. Methazolamide (31) was FDA approved for the treatment of glaucoma, while melatonin (32) inhibited oxygen/glucose deprivation—induced cell death, loss of mitochondrial membrane potential, release of mitochondrial factors, pro-IL-1β processing, and activation of caspase-1 and -3 in primary cerebrocortical neurons. Furthermore, compounds (32, 33) decreased infarct size and improved neurological scores after middle cerebral artery occlusion in mice [54–56]. Gamma-tocotrienol (GTT) (33) had the antiapoptotic effects by preventing the activation of caspase-3 and caspase-9, reducing the release of cytochrome C from the mitochondria and preventing H_2O_2-induced apoptosis in human diploid fibroblasts (HDFs), and delayed cellular aging [57].

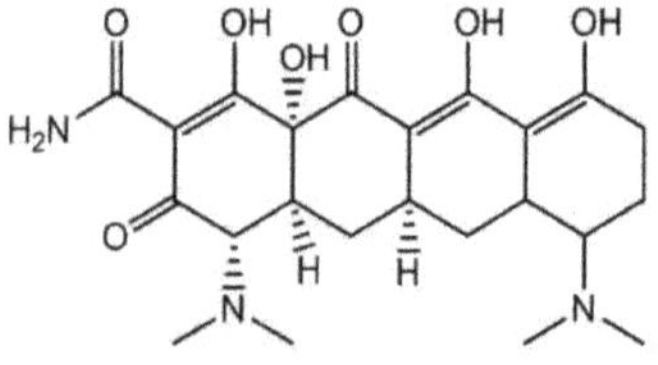

Minocycline
30

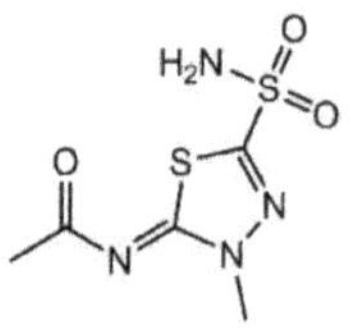

Methazolamide
31

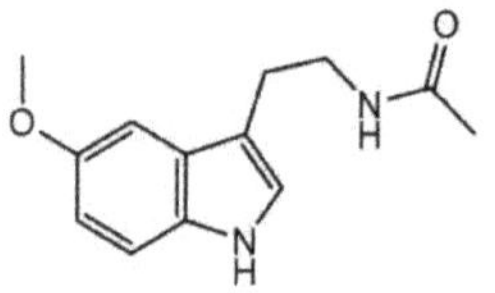

melatonin
32

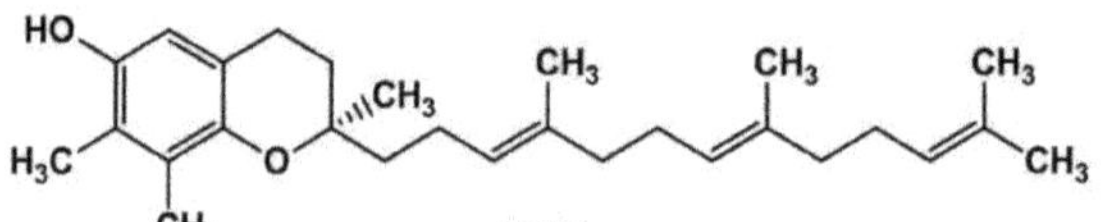

GTT
33

3-hydroxypropyl-triphenylphosphonium (TPP)-conjugated imidazole-substituted oleic acid (TPP-IOA(34a)) and stearic acid (TPP-ISA(34b)) exerted strong specific liganding of heme-iron in cytochrome C/cardiolipin (CL) complex and effectively suppressed its peroxidase activity and CL peroxidation, thus preventing cytochrome C release and cell death, and protecting mice against lethal doses of irradiation [58, 59]. TPP-6-ISA (35) was an effective inhibitor of the peroxidase function of cyt c/CL complexes with a significant antiapoptotic activity that realized in mouse embryonic cells exposed to ionizing irradiation [60, 61].

Tpp-IOA   34a

TPP-ISA   34b

TPP-6-ISA   35

1.2.6 P53 upregulated modulator of apoptosis (PUMA) inhibitors

It is a Bcl-2 homology 3 (BH3)-only Bcl-2 family member and a key mediator of apoptosis induced by a wide variety of stimuli 106. PUMA inhibitors may provide radiation protection and mitigation, there were three compounds that had a strong PUMA inhibition and that were designed by Gabriela Mustata et al., and data were not published due to intellectual property protection [62].

CLZ-8   36

CLZ-8 (36) was capable of targeting a PUMA protein and has very good physicochemical properties, very good apoptosis resistance, and radiation protection effects. It was found to protect cells from DNA damage under the concentration of 1 μm [63].

1.2.7 Bax inhibitors

Xanthan gum (XG) (37) is an extracellular polysaccharide secreted by microorganisms and was first discovered during fermentation process using Xanthomonas campestris. It could protect subchondral trabecular in bone subchondral, decrease the apoptosis of chondrocytes, downregulate the expressions of active caspase-9, active caspase-3 and bax, and upregulate the expression of bcl-2. Lower range of molecular weight of xanthan gum (LRWXG) could upregulate the expression of cytochrome C in mitochondria while downregulating the expression of cytochrome C in cytoplasm. These findings showed that LRWXG could inhibit cartilage degradation via an intrinsic bax-mitochondria cytochrome C-caspase pathway [64].

LRWXG 37

PD98059 (38) showed inhibition of staurosporine-, UV-, anticancer drug-induced apoptosis in vitro and protected brain against cell death through inhibition of BAX and other factors [65, 66]. Vitamin E (39) significantly reduced the effects of gentamicin on BAX and BCL-2 expression levels [67].

Tanshinone (40) could inhibit the expression of Bax and stimulated the expression of Bcl-2 in cardiomyocytes in the ischemia-reperfusion rat model [68].

PD98059 38

Vit.E 39

Tanshinone 40

2. Conclusion

Apoptotic inhibitors regulate cell proliferation by promoting cell survival. One promising area of research that has been covered extensively in this review is displaying the recent developed apoptotic inhibitors and their significance to functional therapies for a number of diseases and pathophysiologies. These inhibitors are working through numerous built-in avenues' mechanisms, including inhibition of pro-apoptotic and apoptotic factors. Our perspectives are to develop new therapeutic strategies aiming to participate in treatment of serious diseases such as stroke, neurodegeneration, retinal cell death, myocardial and liver ischemia, sepsis, osteoarthritis (OA), rheumatoid arthritis (RA), and asthma or to reduce the adverse effects accompanied with long-term therapy of cancer and autoimmunity. Hopefully, scientists will soon be able to provide every patient suffering from imbalanced apoptotic disease with a more specified and suitable therapy.

Conflict of interest

No financial or commercial conflicts of interest were declared by all authors.

Author details

El-Shimaa Mohamed Naguib Abdelhafez[1*], Sara Mohamed Naguib Abdelhafez Ali[2], Mohamed Ramadan Eisa Hassan[3] and Adel Mohammed Abdel-Hakem[1]

1 Department of Medicinal Chemistry, Faculty of Pharmacy, Minia University, Minia, Egypt

2 Department of Histology, Faculty of Medicine, Minia University, Minia, Egypt

3 Department of Organic Chemistry, Faculty of Pharmacy, Azhar University, Egypt

*Address all correspondence to: shimaanaguib_80@mu.edu.eg

IntechOpen

© 2019 The Author(s). Licensee IntechOpen. This chapter is distributed under the terms of the Creative Commons Attribution License (http://creativecommons.org/licenses/by/3.0), which permits unrestricted use, distribution, and reproduction in any medium, provided the original work is properly cited.

References

[1] Guicciardi ME, Gores GJ. Apoptosis: A mechanism of acute and chronic liver injury. Gut. 2005;**54**(7):1024-1033

[2] Portt L, Norman G, Clapp C, Greenwood M, Greenwood MT. Anti-apoptosis and cell survival: A review. Biochimica et Biophysica Acta (BBA)-Molecular Cell Research. 2011;**1813**: 238-259

[3] Ergun U, Yurtcu E, Ergun MA. Protective effect of *Ginkgo biloba* against gossypol-induced apoptosis in human lymphocytes. Cell Biology International. 2005;**29**:717-720

[4] Tian Y-M, Tian H-J, Zhang G-Y, Dai Y-R. Effects of *Ginkgo biloba* extract (EGb 761) on hydroxyl radical-induced thymocyte apoptosis and on age-related thymic atrophy and peripheral immune dysfunctions in mice. Mechanisms of Ageing and Development. 2003;**124**: 977-983

[5] Schindowski K, Leutner S, Kressmann S, Eckert A, Müller WE. Age-related increase of oxidative stress-induced apoptosis in mice prevention by *Ginkgo biloba* extract (EGb761). Journal of Neural Transmission. 2001;**108**: 969-978

[6] Ao Q, Sun X, Wang A, Fu P, Gong K, Zuo H, et al. Protective effects of extract of *Ginkgo biloba* (EGb 761) on nerve cells after spinal cord injury in rats. Spinal Cord. 2006;**44**:662

[7] Rojas P, Serrano-García N, Mares-Sámano JJ, Medina-Campos ON, Pedraza-Chaverri J, Ögren SO. EGb761 protects against nigrostriatal dopaminergic neurotoxicity in 1-methyl-4-phenyl-1, 2, 3, 6-tetrahydropyridine-induced Parkinsonism in mice: Role of oxidative stress. European Journal of Neuroscience. 2008;**28**:41-50

[8] Singh BK, Tripathi M, Chaudhari BP, Pandey PK, Kakkar P. Natural terpenes prevent mitochondrial dysfunction, oxidative stress and release of apoptotic proteins during nimesulide-hepatotoxicity in rats. PLoS ONE. 2012; **7**:e34200

[9] Wang J-m, Qu Z-q, Wu J-l, Chung P, Zeng Y-S. Mitochondrial protective and anti-apoptotic effects of *Rhodiola crenulata* extract on hippocampal neurons in a rat model of Alzheimer's disease. Neural Regeneration Research. 2017;**12**:2025

[10] Charalampopoulos I, Tsatsanis C, Dermitzaki E, Alexaki V-I, Castanas E, Margioris AN, et al. Dehydroepiandrosterone and allopregnanolone protect sympathoadrenal medulla cells against apoptosis via antiapoptotic Bcl-2 proteins. Proceedings of the National Academy of Sciences. 2004;**101**: 8209-8214

[11] Dholakiya SL, Benzeroual KE. Protective effect of diosmin on LPS-induced apoptosis in PC12 cells and inhibition of TNF-α expression. Toxicology in Vitro. 2011;**25**:1039-1044

[12] Danese S. Mechanisms of action of infliximab in inflammatory bowel disease: An anti-inflammatory multitasker. Digestive and Liver Disease. 2008;**40**:S225-S228

[13] Couderc M, Mathieu S, Tournadre A, Dubost J-J, Soubrier M. Acute ocular myositis occurring under etanercept for rheumatoid arthritis. Joint, Bone, Spine. 2014;**81**(5):445-446

[14] Renna S, Mocciaro F, Ventimiglia M, Orlando R, Macaluso FS, Cappello M, et al. A real life comparison of the effectiveness of adalimumab and golimumab in moderate-to-severe

ulcerative colitis, supported by propensity score analysis. Digestive and Liver Disease. [Epub ahead of print]. 2018;**50**:1292-1298

[15] Motlis A, Boktor M, Jordan P, Cvek U, Trutschl M, Alexander JS. Two year follow-up of Crohn's patients substituted to certolizumab anti-TNFα therapy: SAVANT 2. Pathophysiology. 2017;**24**(4):291-295

[16] Chen JJ, Dewdney N, Lin X, Martin RL, Walker KA, Huang J, et al. Design and synthesis of orally active inhibitors of TNF synthesis as anti-rheumatoid arthritis drugs. Bioorganic & Medicinal Chemistry Letters. 2003;**13**(22): 3951-3954

[17] Tweedie D, Luo W, Short RG, Brossi A, Holloway HW, Li Y, et al. A cellular model of inflammation for identifying TNF-α synthesis inhibitors. Journal of Neuroscience Methods. 2009;**183**(2): 182-187

[18] Bhandari P, Patel NK, Gangwal RP, Sangamwar AT, Bhutani KK. Oleanolic acid analogs as NO, TNF-α and IL-1β inhibitors: Synthesis, biological evaluation and docking studies. Bioorganic & Medicinal Chemistry Letters. 2014;**24**(17): 4114-4119

[19] Khalil NA, Ahmed EM, Mohamed KO, Zaitone SA-B. Synthesis of new nicotinic acid derivatives and their evaluation as analgesic and anti-inflammatory agents. Chemical & Pharmaceutical Bulletin. 2013;**61**(9): 933-940

[20] Kumar RS, Antonisamy P, Almansour AI, Arumugam N, Periyasami G, Altaf M, et al. Functionalized spirooxindole-indolizine hybrids: Stereoselective green synthesis and evaluation of anti-inflammatory effect involving TNF-α and nitrite inhibition. European Journal of Medicinal Chemistry. 2018;**15**:2417-2423

[21] Dhuru S, Bhedi D, Gophane D, Hirbhagat K, Nadar V, More D, et al. Novel diarylheptanoids as inhibitors of TNF-α production. Bioorganic & Medicinal Chemistry Letters. 2011; **21**(12):3784-3787

[22] Wang D, Chen P, Chen L, Zeng F, Zang R, Liu H, et al. Betulinic acid protects the neuronal damage in new born rats from isoflurane-induced apoptosis in the developing brain by blocking FASL-FAS signaling pathway. Biomedicine & Pharmacotherapy. 2017; **95**:1631-1635

[23] Yoo S, Yu C, Jung S, Kim E, Kang NS. Design and synthesis of fluorescent and biotin tagged probes for the study of molecular actions of FAF1 inhibitor. Bioorganic & Medicinal Chemistry Letters. 2016;**26**(4):1169-1172

[24] Kakeya H, Miyake Y, Shoji M, Kishida S, Hayashi Y, Kataoka T, et al. Novel non-peptide inhibitors targeting death receptor-mediated apoptosis. Bioorganic & Medicinal Chemistry Letters. 2003;**13**(21):3743-3746

[25] Lu Y, Zhang J, Ma B, Li K, Li X, Bai H, et al. Glycine attenuates cerebral ischemia/reperfusion injury by inhibiting neuronal apoptosis in mice. Neurochemistry International. 2012; **61**(5):649-658

[26] Suh J, Yi KY, Lee Y-S, Kim E, Yum EK, Yoo S. Synthesis and biological evaluation of 3-substituted-benzofuran-2-carboxylic esters as a novel class of ischemic cell death inhibitors. Bioorganic & Medicinal Chemistry Letters. 2010;**20**(22):6362-6365

[27] Li Q, Nakadai A, Takeda K, Kawada T. Dimethyl 2,2-dichlorovinyl phosphate (DDVP) markedly inhibits activities of natural killer cells, cytotoxic

T lymphocytes and lymphokine-activated killer cells via the Fas-ligand/Fas pathway in perforin-knockout (PKO) mice. Toxicology. 2004;**204**(1): 41-50

[28] He W, Wu L, Gao Q, Du Y, Wang Y. Identification of AHBA biosynthetic genes related to geldanamycin biosynthesis in *Streptomyces hygroscopicus* 17997. Current Microbiology. 2006;**52**(3):197-203

[29] Yin X-H, Han Y-L, Zhuang Y, Yan J-Z, Li C. Geldanamycin inhibits Fas signaling pathway and protects neurons against ischemia. Neuroscience Research. 2017;**12**:433-439

[30] Duque G, El Abdaimi K, Henderson JE, Lomri A, Kremer R. Vitamin D inhibits Fas ligand-induced apoptosis in human osteoblasts by regulating components of both the mitochondrial and Fas-related pathways. Bone. 2004; **35**(1):57-64

[31] Jia J, Guan D, Zhu W, Alkayed NJ, Wang MM, Hua Z, et al. Estrogen inhibits Fas-mediated apoptosis in experimental stroke. Experimental Neurology. 2009;**215**(1): 48-52

[32] Xie Z, Koyama T, Abe K. Effects of an angiotensin-converting enzyme inhibitor on the expression of Fas protein and on apoptosis in rat ventricles subjected to reperfusion after ischemia. Current Therapeutic Research. 2000;**61**(6):358-366

[33] Tsuda T, Ohmori Y, Muramatsu H, Hosaka Y, Takiguchi K, Saitoh F, et al. Inhibitory effect of M50054, a novel inhibitor of apoptosis, on anti-Fas-antibody-induced hepatitis and chemotherapy-induced alopecia. European Journal of Pharmacology. 2001;**433**(1):37-45

[34] Liu W, Jing Z-T, Wu S-X, He Y, Lin Y-T, Chen W-N, et al. Novel AKT activator, SC79, prevents acute hepatic failure induced by Fas-mediated apoptosis of hepatocytes. The American Journal of Pathology. 2018;**188**(5): 1171-1182

[35] Urayama S, Kawakami A, Nakashima T, Tsuboi M, Yamasaki S, Hida A, et al. Effect of vitamin K2 on osteoblast apoptosis: Vitamin K2 inhibits apoptotic cell death of human osteoblasts induced by Fas, proteasome inhibitor, etoposide, and staurosporine. Journal of Laboratory and Clinical Medicine. 2000;**136**(3):181-193

[36] Stanely Mainzen Prince P, Dhanasekar K, Rajakumar S. Vanillic acid prevents altered ion pumps, ions, inhibits Fas-receptor and caspase mediated apoptosis-signaling pathway and cardiomyocyte death in myocardial infarcted rats. Chemico-Biological Interactions. 2015;**23**:268-276

[37] Fiorucci S, Mencarelli A, Palazzetti B, Del Soldato P, Morelli A, Ignarro LJ. An NO derivative of ursodeoxycholic acid protects against Fas-mediated liver injury by inhibiting caspase activity. Proceedings of the National Academy of Sciences of the United States of America. 2001;**98**(5):2652-2657

[38] Adrain C, Creagh EM, Martin SJ. Apoptosis-associated release of Smac/DIABLO from mitochondria requires active caspases and is blocked by Bcl-2. The EMBO Journal. 2001;**20**(23): 6627-6636

[39] Becattini B, Sareth S, Zhai D, Crowell KJ, Leone M, Reed JC, et al. Targeting apoptosis via chemical design: Inhibition of bid-induced cell death by small organic molecules. Chemistry & Biology. 2004;**11**(8):1107-1117

[40] Yuan J. Neuroprotective strategies targeting apoptotic and necrotic cell death for stroke. Apoptosis. 2009;**14**(4): 469-477

[41] Martin NA, Bonner H, Elkjær ML, D'Orsi B, Chen G, König HG, et al. BID mediates oxygen-glucose deprivation-induced neuronal injury in organotypic hippocampal slice cultures and modulates tissue inflammation in a transient focal cerebral ischemia model without changing lesion volume. Frontiers in Cellular Neuroscience; Feb 3 2016;**10**:14. DOI: 10.3389/fncel.2016.00014

[42] Brenner C, Galluzzi L, Kepp O, Kroemer G. Decoding cell death signals in liver inflammation. Journal of Hepatology. 2013;**59**(3):583-594

[43] Wang C, Youle RJ. The role of mitochondria in apoptosis. Annual Review of Genetics. 2009;**43**:95-118

[44] Li L, Jiang X, Huang S, Ying Z, Zhang Z, Pan C, et al. Discovery of highly potent 2-sulfonyl-pyrimidinyl derivatives for apoptosis inhibition and ischemia treatment. ACS Medicinal Chemistry Letters. 2017;**8**(4):407-412

[45] Becattini B, Culmsee C, Leone M, Zhai D, Zhang X, Crowell KJ, et al. Structure–activity relationships by interligand NOE-based design and synthesis of antiapoptotic compounds targeting bid. Proceedings of the National Academy of Sciences of the United States of America. 2006;**103**(33):12602-12606

[46] Oppermann S, Schrader FC, Elsässer K, Dolga AM, Kraus AL, Doti N, et al. Novel N-phenyl–substituted thiazolidinediones protect neural cells against glutamate- and tBid-induced toxicity. The Journal of Pharmacology and Experimental Therapeutics. 2014;**350**(2):273-289

[47] Maecker H, Varfolomeev E, Kischkel F, Lawrence D, LeBlanc H, Lee W, et al. TWEAK attenuates the transition from innate to adaptive immunity. Cell. 2005;**123**(5):931-944

[48] Wajant H. The TWEAK-Fn14 system as a potential drug target. British Journal of Pharmacology. 2013;**170**(4):748-764

[49] Roos A, Dhruv HD, Mathews IT, Inge LJ, Tuncali S, Hartman LK, et al. Identification of aurintricarboxylic acid as a selective inhibitor of the TWEAK-Fn14 signaling pathway in glioblastoma cells. Oncotarget. 2017;**8**(7):12234-12246

[50] Tran N, Meurice N, Dhruv H. FN14 antagonists and therapeutic uses thereof. 2016. US9238034B2

[51] Dhruv H, Loftus JC, Narang P, Petit JL, Fameree M, Burton J, et al. Structural basis and targeting of the interaction between fibroblast growth factor-inducible 14 and tumor necrosis factor-like weak inducer of apoptosis. The Journal of Biological Chemistry. 2013;**288**(45):32261-32276

[52] Maneg O, Malatesta F, Ludwig B, Drosou V. Interaction of cytochrome C with cytochrome oxidase: Two different docking scenarios. Biochimica et Biophysica Acta (BBA)-Bioenergetics. 2004;**1655**:274-281

[53] Zhu S, Stavrovskaya IG, Drozda M, Kim BYS, Ona V, Li M, et al. Minocycline inhibits cytochrome C release and delays progression of amyotrophic lateral sclerosis in mice. Nature. 2002;**417**(6884):74-78

[54] Wang X, Zhu S, Pei Z, Drozda M, Stavrovskaya IG, Del Signore SJ, et al. Inhibitors of cytochrome C release with therapeutic potential for Huntington's disease. The Journal of Neuroscience. 2008;**28**(38):9473-9485

[55] Wang X, Figueroa BE, Stavrovskaya IG, Zhang Y, Sirianni AC, Zhu S, et al. Methazolamide and melatonin inhibit mitochondrial cytochrome C release and are neuroprotective in experimental models of ischemic injury. Stroke. [Epub ahead of print]. 2009;**14**:1877-1885

[56] Li M, Wang W, Mai H, Zhang X, Wang J, Gao Y, et al. Methazolamide improves neurological behavior by inhibition of neuron apoptosis in subarachnoid hemorrhage mice. Scientific Reports. 2016;6:35055

[57] Makpol S, Abdul Rahim N, Kien Hui C, Ngah W, Zurinah W. Inhibition of mitochondrial cytochrome C release and suppression of caspases by gamma-tocotrienol prevent apoptosis and delay aging in stress-induced premature senescence of skin fibroblasts. Oxidative Medicine and Cellular Longevity. 2012; **2012**:1-13. Available from: https://www.hindawi.com/journals/omcl/2012/785743/ [Accessed: September 24, 2018]

[58] Atkinson J, Kapralov AA, Yanamala N, Tyurina YY, Amoscato AA, Pearce L, et al. A mitochondria-targeted inhibitor of cytochrome C peroxidase mitigates radiation-induced death. Nature Communications. 2011;**2**:497

[59] Bakan A, Kapralov AA, Bayir H, Hu F, Kagan VE, Bahar I. Inhibition of peroxidase activity of cytochrome C: De novo compound discovery and validation. Molecular Pharmacology. 2015;**88**(3):421-427

[60] Jiang J, Bakan A, Kapralov AA, Silva KI, Huang Z, Amoscato AA, et al. Designing inhibitors of cytochrome C/cardiolipin peroxidase complexes: Mitochondria-targeted imidazole-substituted fatty acids. Free Radical Biology & Medicine. 2014;**71**:221-230

[61] Ghosh AP, Walls KC, Klocke BJ, Toms R, Strasser A, Roth KA. The pro-apoptotic BH3-only, Bcl-2 family member Puma is critical for acute ethanol-induced neuronal apoptosis. Journal of Neuropathology and Experimental Neurology. 2009;**68**(7):747-756

[62] Mustata G, Li M, Zevola N, Bakan A, Zhang L, Epperly M, et al. Development of small-molecule PUMA inhibitors for mitigating radiation-induced cell death. Current Topics in Medicinal Chemistry. 2011;**11**(3):281-290

[63] Feng T, Liu J, Zhou N, Wang L, Liu X, Zhang S, et al. CLZ-8, a potent small-molecular compound, protects radiation-induced damages both in vitro and in vivo. Environmental Toxicology and Pharmacology. 2018;**61**:44-51

[64] Shao X, Chen Q, Dou X, Chen L, Wu J, Zhang W, et al. Lower range of molecular weight of xanthan gum inhibits cartilage matrix destruction via intrinsic bax-mitochondria cytochrome C-caspase pathway. Carbohydrate Polymers. 2018;**198**:354-363

[65] Sawatzky DA, Willoughby DA, Colville-Nash PR, Rossi AG. The involvement of the apoptosis-modulating proteins ERK 1/2, Bcl-xL and Bax in the resolution of acute inflammation in vivo. The American Journal of Pathology. 2006;**168**(1):33-41

[66] Nguyen Thi PA, Chen M-H, Li N, Zhuo X-J, Xie L. PD98059 protects brain against cells death resulting from ROS/ERK activation in a cardiac arrest rat model. Oxidative Medicine and Cellular Longevity. 2016;**2016**:3723762. Available from: https://www.hindawi.com/journals/omcl/2016/3723762/ [Accessed: December 10, 2018]

[67] Kandeil MAM, Hassanin KMA, Mohammed ET, Safwat GM, Mohamed DS. Wheat germ and vitamin E decrease BAX/BCL-2 ratio in rat kidney treated with gentamicin. Beni-Suef University Journal of Basic and Applied Sciences. 2018;7(3):257-262

[68] Guo R, Li G. Tanshinone modulates the expression of Bcl-2 and Bax in cardiomyocytes and has a protective effect in a rat model of myocardial ischemia-reperfusion. Hellenic Journal of Cardiology. [Epub ahead of print]. 2018;**59**:323-328

Section 2

Methods in Cytotoxicity Assessment

Chapter 6

Cell Division, Cytotoxicity, and the Assays Used in the Detection of Cytotoxicity

Erman Salih Istifli, Mehmet Tahir Hüsunet and Hasan Basri Ila

Abstract

Cell division is a phenomenon that is encountered in all cells in nature. While normal cell division results in proliferation in single-celled organisms, and development and repair in multicellular organisms, aberrant and untimely cell division results in tumor formation. Therefore, the understanding of the cell division is hidden in identifying the details of the molecular mechanisms that govern cellular division at the exact time and under right conditions. Sometimes these molecular mechanisms are distorted by both intrinsic and extracellular factors, and the division process halts or deviates to an abnormal pathway. At this point, it is essential that the abnormal cells are removed from the tissue by an appropriate mechanism. In this context, in this review, general and specific information about cell division and its molecular control mechanisms were discussed, and different types of cell death mechanisms were mentioned accordingly. In addition, chemical, biological, and physical cytotoxic agents that negatively affect cell division and their mechanisms of action are explained. Finally, a brief review of the principles of different cytotoxicity (cell viability and proliferation) test systems has been performed to provide a source of information for investigators who study cell viability, proliferation, or different types of cellular death pathways.

Keywords: cell division, DNA damage, cell cycle control, mutagens, cellular proliferation parameters, cytotoxicity assays

1. Introduction

Cell division is a common phenomenon that occurs in all living entities, except for cells that have completed somatic differentiation. When the cell reaches a certain volume, it performs division [1]. While the cell division leads to an increase in the number of individuals in single-celled organisms, in multicellular organisms, it ensures the growth of hair and nails, healing of wounds, cellular repair, somatic growth, and genesis of reproductive cells. Then, one might question that under what conditions do cells divide? Before moving on to the answer for this question, it is crucial to find the answer to this proposal: **Do cells divide because they grow? Or do they grow because they need to be divided?** The various assumptions about the view that advocates the premise that the cell divides because it grows are summarized below:

1. **Overall control attenuates as the cell grows.** Later in the process of cell growth, obstacles start to appear in the central management of the organelles in the cytoplasm. As a result, problems may arise in the way organelles perform their tasks and also in the control of the communication they perform with each other. In addition, the material exchange within the cell starts to become inextricable [2]. In summary, since the growth of the cell will cause a number of significant difficulties in performing intracellular coordination activities, the cell needs divisions to reduce its volume.

2. **As the cell grows, the "cytoplasm/nucleus" ratio varies in favor of the cytoplasm.** Since the increase in volume of the cytoplasm makes it difficult for the nucleus to maintain its control on the cell, it is crucial for cell to divide and restore the optimal cytoplasm/nucleus ratio [3].

3. **Since the cell membrane does not enlarge as fast as the cytoplasm, it becomes difficult for the cell to exchange material from the external environment during continuous cell growth.** To achieve sufficient material exchange from the membranes, the membrane-to-surface area must reach the optimum value [4]. As the cell continues to grow, difficulties in maintaining the surface-volume balance begin. Small or thin objects have a larger surface area than their volume. This gives them a large surface-to-volume ratio. However, large objects have a small surface area than their volume; thus they have a small surface-to-volume ratio [1].

This could be best explained by a balloon blowing event. As a balloon swells, the internal volume increases, but the membrane cannot simultaneously compensate for this volume increase and, thus, explodes after a certain time period. Cells need to divide to prevent this negative event (otherwise, cells would become lysed).

4. **Environmental factors and hormones can lead the cell to division.** In general, if any tissue has been damaged for any reason, cell division takes place and performs the repair process. In this context, growth hormone may be given as an example of the effect of hormones on cell division. These and similar hormones have mitogenic functions that trigger a cell division signal [5–7].

In fact, from a scientific point of view, the cell is divided not because it grows, but rather it requires division. In the process of cell division, the dividing cell is called a parental or host cell. The parental cell is divided into two daughter cells. Subsequent divisions are then repeated via the so-called process, the cell cycle.

Cells regulate the division process by communicating with each other through chemical signals generated by specific proteins called cyclin and cyclin-dependent kinases [8]. These signals play a key role in determining when cells will begin to divide and stop dividing. Cell division is important for the growth of the organism and wound healing. It is also important that the cells terminate dividing at the appropriate time [9]. Otherwise, cancer occurs because the cells do not stop the division at the required time.

Cells in the organism perform division for growth and/or repair; on the one hand, they undergo apoptosis (by cellular turnover) for various reasons to maintain homeostasis. Because some cells, such as epidermal cells, are constantly lost, new cells must be produced via cell division. For instance, 30,000–40,000 epidermal cells are killed per minute by apoptosis [10]. In other words, we lose about 50 million cells each day. Therefore, cell division is very important in tissues where cells are lost very rapidly. However, other cells such as the nerve cells are either not divided or very rarely divided [11].

Depending on the cell type, cell division has two mechanisms: mitosis and meiosis. Each of these cell division mechanisms has unique characteristics. In mitosis, the parent cell (diploid, 2n) is divided into two daughter cells with the identical number of chromosomes [12]. This type of cell division is essential for basic growth and repair. On the other hand, the parental cell in meiosis (diploid, 2n) is divided into four cells with two successive cleavages (meiosis I and meiosis II), and the number of chromosomes are half the main cell (haploid, n) [13]. The reduction of the diploid chromosome number to haploid is important for sexual reproduction, and recombination in meiosis I is the source of genetic diversity.

The cell, which has not yet started to divide, is in the interphase of the cell cycle. Cells have to be divided by certain periods, though each cell actually passes most of its time in the interphase. The interphase is the period when a cell is prepared to divide and initiate the cell cycle [14]. During this time, the cells have to obtain nutrients and energy. The host cell also synthesizes a copy of its DNA to share equally between the two daughter cells.

However, if cell division is not required for the functional integrity of the organism, negative regulation of the cell cycle is performed [15]. In contrast to the positive regulators, the negative regulators function in a direction that halts the cell cycle. In this process, a large number of molecular components and signaling are involved. The most well-studied negative regulatory molecules are the retinoblastoma protein (Rb), p53, and p21 [16]. These three proteins have been commonly referred as tumor suppressor proteins. Like the p53 and p21 proteins, Rb proteins are also a group of tumor suppressor proteins observed in many cell types. Most of the knowledge of cell cycle regulation have been obtained from studies using cells that have lost control of cell cycle regulation [17–19]. It has been discovered that cells that are uncontrolled (becoming cancerous) have these regulatory proteins damaged or nonfunctional [20, 21]. In each case, the major cause of uncontrolled progression through the cell cycle is errors in the abovementioned regulatory proteins. In this case, the possibility of uncontrolled cellular proliferation is raised. When DNA damage is detected, p53 protein halts the cell cycle and DNA repair enzymes are activated to repair the damage. However, if DNA damage cannot be repaired, the p53 protein may trigger apoptosis (programmed cell suicide) to prevent the replication of damaged chromosomes [22]. Different cellular death pathways including apoptosis, in the context of this chapter, are therefore summarized below.

2. General mechanisms of cell death

2.1 Apoptosis

Apoptosis, also known as programmed cell death, is a regulated cellular destruction program that facilitates the removal of damaged or excess cells. This process is critical for many physiological processes including embryonic development and tissue homeostasis in adulthood [23, 24].

Multicellular organisms have developed suppressive processes that prevent the proliferation of cells displaying aberrant proliferation or improper tissue infiltration. These processes function to block tissue hyperplasia, tumor formation, and metastatic distribution of tumors. Processes such as the cell cycle arrest, cellular aging, and apoptotic cell death, which remove malicious cells capable of initiating tumor growth, can also be included in this mechanism [25].

2.2 Autophagy

Autophagy (or autophagocytosis) (autóphagos in Ancient Greek) means "self-devouring." It is the natural regulating mechanism that extracts the nonfunctional (junk) components of the cell [26]. The term "autophagy" was first used in 1963 by the Belgian biochemist Christian de Duve [27]. In the 1990s, the Japanese autophagy researcher Yoshinori Ohsumi discovered the mechanisms of autophagy in yeast cell by identification of autophagy genes and received the 2016 Nobel Prize in Physiology and Medicine for his studies [28]. Autophagy allows the regular degradation and recycling of cellular components [29]. The cytoplasmic components targeted in this pathway are separated by a double-membrane vesicle named autophagosome from the rest of the cell [30, 31]. The autophagosome then fuses with the lysosome and performs the digestion of the cellular components in between its membranes. In general, three types of autophagy have been reported to date, including macro- and microautophagy and chaperone-mediated autophagy. Although the autophagic process, in the context of the disease, was observed to be an adaptive stress response that increases survival, it has been observed in other cases that it increased cell death and morbidity. In the case of excessive cellular starvation, disintegration of cellular components promotes survival by ensuring that cellular energy levels remain constant [32]. Autophagy, which acts as a protective response to biological stress in mammalian cells, removes damaged proteins and organelles from the cytoplasm and allows for the reconstitution of components in their structure using lysosomal content. In the case of moderate stress, autophagy may undertake the task of survival; however, in the event of excessive stress, it can activate the programmed cell death pathway [33]. Because of the dysregulation of autophagy in many diseases including cancer, it is crucial to understand how the transition from autophagy to apoptosis occurs. Cells that respond to exogenous stress were found to be consistent in their quantitative autophagy and apoptosis measurements [34]. On the other hand, defective apoptosis in immortalized epithelial cells renders cells substantially tumorigenic. In apoptosis-defective cells, activation of AKT (protein kinase B) or allelic degradation of Beclin1 inhibits a pathway of survival due to autophagy, thereby enhancing susceptibility to metabolic stress. Although autophagy acts as a buffer against metabolic stress, the simultaneous disruption of apoptosis and autophagy mechanism promotes necrotic cell death in vitro and in vivo. Therefore, the inhibition of autophagy by certain conditions, such as nutrient starvation, may render apoptosis-resistant tumors susceptible to apoptosis [35]. While apoptosis acts as a cellular quality control mechanism in the organism, autophagy acts as an intracellular quality control mechanism. Collectively, autophagy and apoptosis are not interchangeable metabolic pathways, and autophagy can be assumed as one of the components of apoptosis.

2.3 Necrosis

Another pathway of cell death is necrotic cell death. Necrosis (Greek: death) is a form of cell injury that results in premature death of cells in living tissues through the mechanism of autolysis [36]. Necrosis is caused by factors other than cells or tissues, such as infection, toxins, or trauma, which cause irregular digestion of cell components. Unlike apoptosis, it is not a controlled or programmed type of death. Apoptosis is often beneficial to the organism, while necrosis is almost always disastrous and may be fatal [37]. Cell death from necrosis does not follow the path of apoptotic signaling, but more diverse receptors are activated, resulting in loss of cell membrane integrity and uncontrolled release of cell death products into the extracellular domain [36]. This initiates an inflammatory response in the surrounding tissue that activates leukocytes and nearby phagocytes and eliminates dead cells by phagocytosis. However, microbial damaging agents released by leukocytes can cause irreparable damage to the surrounding tissues from the lateral side [38]. There are six different models of necrosis recognized morphologically. These include coagulative necrosis, liquefactive necrosis, gangrenous necrosis, caseous necrosis, fat necrosis, and fibrinoid necrosis [39].

2.4 Necroptosis

Necroptosis is a programmed necrosis or inflammatory cell death pattern. Conventionally, necroptosis, unlike regularly programmed cell death by apoptosis, is associated with non-programmed cell death resulting from cellular damage or infiltration of pathogens. The discovery of necroptosis has shown that cells are capable of performing necrosis in a programmed manner and that apoptosis is not always the only preferred form of cell death [40].

3. Cytotoxicity

The effect of being toxic to cells caused by toxic agents is called cytotoxicity. Exposing cells to a cytotoxic compound may result in various outcomes in the cell. At this point, the cells may actively progress into the death phase. Furthermore, the cells may activate the controlled cell death (apoptosis) program, or necrosis may occur where the membrane integrity is lost and uncontrolled death is being executed due to cell lysis. Cells undergoing the process of necrosis commonly swell rapidly, lose membrane integrity, stop metabolism, and secrete their contents into the extracellular space. Furthermore, cells with rapid necrosis in vitro do not have enough time or energy to initiate apoptotic mechanisms and therefore will not express apoptotic indicators. Apoptosis is characterized by well-defined cytological and molecular events involving cytoplasmic shrinkage, nuclear condensation, and controlled cleavage of DNA by the endonucleases. Cells in culture undergoing apoptosis eventually undergo secondary necrosis. At this time, the cell stops metabolism and loses the integrity of its membrane [41].

Cytotoxic agents are known as all the elements that are toxic to the cells, which include the factors that prevent their growth and sometimes cause death, and are also used to treat certain disorders. Chemical and biological substances or physical agents can cause cytotoxicity by affecting the cells in varying degrees. These agents include chemical agents that act by inhibiting synthesis (such as nucleic acid and protein synthesis) in the cell, by affecting cellular energy production pathways (mitochondrial effect), or by attenuating the integrity of the membrane in the cell (plasma membrane or intracellular organelles that have membranes).

3.1 Chemical cytotoxic agents (cytostatics)

- Inhibitors of dihydrofolate reductase responsible for purine and pyrimidine biosynthesis.

- Inhibitors of DNA biosynthesis (cytarabine).

- DNA intercalators (anthracyclines and anthracenediones).

- Agents inducing DNA strand break formation (bleomycin).

- DNA topoisomerase inhibitors (camptothecin, anthracyclines, anthracenediones, anthrapyrazole, and etoposide).

- Cytotoxic agents that cause formation of DNA adducts (cyclophosphamide, melphalan, chlorambucil, hexamethylmelamine, busulfan, dacarbazine, mitomycin C, and cisplatin).

- RNA degradation (inhibition of RNA biosynthesis by anthracyclines).

- Nucleoprotein (inhibition of nucleoprotein synthesis by L-asparaginase) and microtubule biosynthesis inhibitors (antitubulin, colchicine, dolastatin, taxol, tritlisin, vinblastine, and vincristine).

- Agents that cause cytotoxicity by modulating the mitochondrial permeability transition pores and increasing the mitochondrial membrane potential and affecting the energy transmission pathways in neoplastic cells. These agents include staurosporine, poly (ADP-ribose) polymerase, 6-aminonicotinamide, 6-methyl-mercaptopurine ribid, 6-mercaptopurinoside, 6-aminonicotinamide and 6-methyl-mercaptopurinoside, and N- (phosphonacetyl)-L-aspartic acid [42].

3.2 Biological cytotoxic agents

In this group, toxic molecules derived from viruses, bacteria, fungi, plant, and animal origin are generally included. Bacterial endo-/exotoxins and antibiotics in this group are the most widely recognized molecules. Biological agents such as lipid hydrolyzing enzymes, sphingomyelinases C and D, cholesterol oxidase, helianthus toxin, streptolysin, and saponin damaged cultured human skin fibroblasts and erythrocytes with different cholesterol levels. However, erythrocytes with high cholesterol levels were found to be more sensitive to toxins [43]. Cytotoxic agents used by invertebrates include oxygen and nitrogen reactive intermediates, antimicrobial peptides, lectins, cytokines, and quinoid intermediates of melanin [44]. It has also been found that bacterial cytotoxins act by targeting the actin components of the cell skeleton of eukaryotic cells [45].

3.3 Physical cytotoxic agents

Physical agents such as heat, ultrasonic vibrations, and radiation have cytotoxic effects. The toxicity induced by "lethal heat shock" in *Saccharomyces cerevisiae* (yeast) cells was found to be primarily due to oxidative stress. The possibility that mitochondrial membrane disruption in aerobic cells exposed to heat stress is hundreds of times higher than cells in anaerobic conditions reinforcing this possibility [46]. An in vitro study of Chinese hamster ovarian (CHO) cells revealed that the cytotoxicity of drugs affecting the plasma membrane was synergistically increased by ultrasound application [47]. It has also been found that the use of ultrasonic microbubble increases the cytotoxic effects of chemotherapeutic drugs on tumor cells [48]. In addition, many studies in the literature on the cytotoxic effect of radiation can be found.

4. Universal cytotoxicity parameters

Assays to measure the reduction in the cell viability (inhibition of growth/division or death by apoptotic-necrotic pathways) are called "cytotoxicity" tests. These experiments can be performed by in vitro and/or in vivo test systems in different cell types using various techniques. While some of these parameters (mitotic index, replication index, nuclear division index, etc.) contribute to the indirect demonstration of cell division dynamics, some of them directly contribute to the demonstration of cell viability (MTT, MTS, XTT, WST, etc.) [49]. A brief summary of these methods can be found below; however, before explaining these test methods, brief information about some of the most commonly used cytotoxicity parameters that provide us quantitative information about the different cellular processes will be discussed.

4.1 Mitotic index

The mitotic index of a cell population is expressed as a proportion of the population at any mitotic stage (e.g., per mille = 1/1000). Mitotic index is an important criterion for the growth and multiplication of tissues. Because it is calculated in fixed and stained cell preparations at a particular divisional phase, the mitotic index reflects only the division stages of cells at the time of fixation [50]. Furthermore, since cell division is a process that follows DNA replication under normal conditions, the mitotic index is indirectly a parameter that is also associated with DNA replication. One can ask: why has mitotic index attracted considerable interest as a viability parameter for decades in genotoxicity tests? The answer to this question clearly lies in cell division. A successful cell division requires coordination between different cell cycle checkpoints, especially G1/S and G2/M transitions [51]. These cell cycle control points, which regulate the sequence and timing of sub-phase transitions, are essential in maintaining genomic integrity and in realizing a healthy cell division [52]. Therefore, no matter what type of cell is being examined under the microscope, the MI is a universal parameter capable of giving information indirectly about all the subcomponents and control points of the cell cycle and is used to measure cytotoxicity in living organisms. The calculation of MI shows minor differences between plant and animal cells. In plant and animal cells, the MI is simply calculated as follows and is given in percentage:

Plant cells:

$$MI = \frac{Prophase + Metaphase + Anaphase + Telophase}{Total\ number\ of\ cells} \times 100 \qquad (1)$$

Animal cells:

$$MI = \frac{Metaphase\ cells}{Total\ number\ of\ cells} \times 100 \qquad (2)$$

For the calculation of MI in animal cells, the reason for counting only the cells in the metaphase stage is the use of special chemicals (e.g., colchicine, vincristine, vinblastine) that inhibit microtubule polymerization in the metaphase stage during mitosis. Therefore, the cell cannot proceed further than the metaphase stage.

Although not always, a significant decrease in MI correlates with genotoxicity. A reduction of MI by 50% or less indicates a lethal effect on the cells, and this is called lethal dose of 50 [53]. The decline in mitotic index may be related to inhibition of DNA synthesis or delay/stop in cell cycle phases (G1, S, or G2). Occasionally, there may be also significant increases in MI compared to control. This may be due to a reduction in the duration devoted to DNA repair [54] or the acceleration of the transition between the phases of the cell cycle [55]. Both events can result in an uncontrolled progression of cell proliferation.

In recent years, a new formula of mitotic index has been developed which takes account of only actively dividing cells. According to this hypothesis, only actively dividing cells, i.e., metaphase and anaphase cells, are included in the calculation. This formula (active mitotic index) provides additional information on the percentage of actively dividing cells [56, 57]:

$$AMI = \frac{Metaphase + Anaphase}{Total\ number\ of\ cells\ observed} \quad (3)$$

Another characteristic of the MI is that it provides critical information about the progression of the disease and the course of treatment in certain diseases such as cancer. Since one of the hallmarks of cancer is a high rate of cell proliferation, MI can therefore be used as an important predictor in the prognosis of various types of cancer. In this context, high levels of MI were associated with hepatocellular carcinoma (HCC) and invasive breast carcinoma, while low MI values were associated with negative node status, diploid DNA content, low S-phase fraction, and positive estrogen (ER) and progesterone (PgR) receptor status in breast cancer [58–60].

4.2 Nuclear division index (NDI)

Such as the mitotic index, nuclear division index is a parameter that provides information about the numerical value of cell proliferation. The difference of NDI from MI is that NDI is calculated based on the number of nuclei in divided (or interphase) cells. Thus, NDI is a parameter that is directly related with the DNA replication. NDI may be used to gain quantitative information on cell cycle progression of the lymphocytes after phytohaemagglutinin (PHA) stimulation. This index is frequently employed as a useful research tool for understanding the kinetics of cell cycling in lymphocyte cultures. However, although it is simply a tool to measure the rate of division in viable cells, an increase in cell death via necrosis or apoptosis does not always cause a reduction of the NDI in surviving cells [61]. On the other hand, it has been experimentally shown that NDI was associated with various malignancies and could be used as a screening strategy as a cytogenetic biomarker in cancer such as the MI. It has been reported that the mean NDI values were significantly lower in patients with colorectal cancer (CRC) or polyps than in patients with normal colonoscopy. Therefore, NDI was proven to be useful in screening strategies for CRC [62]. The NDI is calculated as in the following formula:

$$NDI = \frac{(M1) + (2 \times M2) + (3 \times M3) + (4 \times M4)}{N} \quad (4)$$

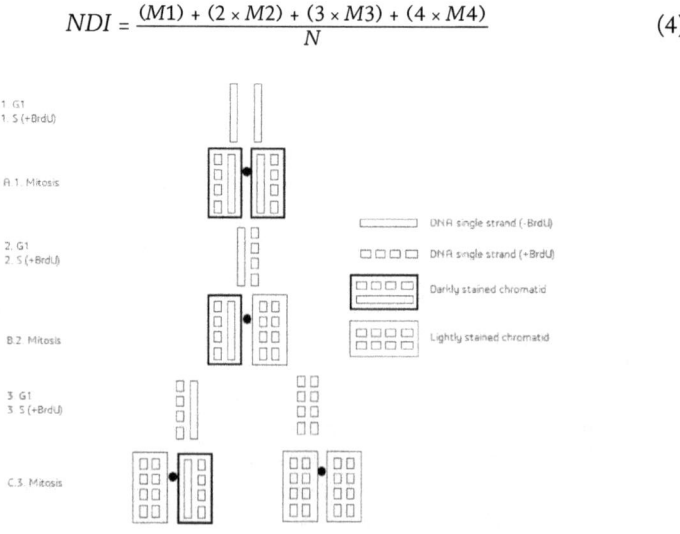

Figure 1.
Schematic representation of the differentiation of cells undergoing the first, second, and third mitotic division with the introduction of BrdU into DNA molecule.

where M1–M4 represent the number of cells with one to four nuclei and N is the total number of the cells scored [63].

4.3 Proliferation index (replication index, BrdU incorporation)

Proliferation index (PI) or replication index (RI) is a parameter that is used to investigate the rate of DNA replication. It is basically a method based on the principle of integration of BrdU into the strands of DNA. BrdU, deoxythymidine (dT), and deoxyuridine (dU) are molecules which are analogues of each other. The difference between these molecules is due to the fact that the chemical groups bound to the fifth C atom in the heterocyclic benzene ring are different (**Figure 1**).

5. In vitro cytotoxicity (cell viability) assays

Before proceeding with the widely used in vitro cytotoxicity tests, it is worth mentioning why these tests are more preferred than animal tests:

1. Although animal tests can provide pathological information, these tests have ethical concerns.

2. In vitro tests conducted in a test tube using cells grown from an organ can be used to test the toxic effects of substances on specific tissues.

3. In vitro tests enable us to screen minimal quantities of chemicals.

4. It could be also possible to study specific subcellular pathways such as signaling pathways and oxidative stress.

However, despite these advantages offered, in vitro cytotoxicity assays cannot fully substitute in vivo assays because:

1. The chemicals may be metabolized inside the whole body rather than specific organs.

2. In vivo tests can be conducted lifelong.

3. In vivo tests enable us to determine the presence of chemicals in multiple organs and their distribution in the body as a whole.

4. Specific systems such as the reproductive system and respiratory system can be examined in vivo.

5. Different routes of entry such as the skin, inhalation, and gut can be tested in vivo.

6. In vivo tests enable us to calculate and model toxicokinetic effects, in terms of uptake and removal, and the half-life of the chemical in the body.

Cytotoxicity tests are among the first in vitro bioassays used to predict toxicity of various substances in different tissues. The need for safety assessment of drugs, cosmetics, food additives, pesticides, and industrial chemicals increases year by year. **Figure 2** demonstrates an overview of the compartments which are targeted by the cytotoxicity test systems within the cell.

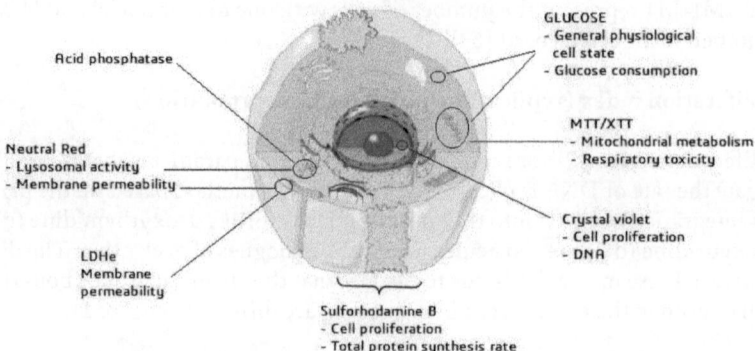

Figure 2.
Overview of general targets of cytotoxicity test systems in the cell.

According to their targeted compartments in the cell, in vitro cytotoxicity assay methods could measure viability or toxicity basically in four different ways: (I) proliferation (direct viable cell count), (II) cell division (DNA synthesis by ^{3}H thymidine uptake), (III) metabolism (MTT, alamar blue, ATP production), and (IV) membrane (leakage of lactate dehydrogenase from dead cells). However, many cytotoxicity tests, although they differ from each other in practice, allow testing of relatively similar cellular processes and endpoints. Therefore, these tests, below, are summarized without dividing into different categories.

5.1 Apoptosis assay

Apoptotic cells are recognized by reduced DNA content and morphological changes such as nuclear condensation that can be detectable by flow cytometry, trypan blue, or Hoechst staining. Changes in the structure and function of the plasma membrane are determined by the appearance of phosphatidylserine on the plasma membrane that reacts with the Annexin V-fluorochrome conjugates. Propidium iodide (PI) staining allows distinction between early and late apoptotic events [64].

5.2 ATP assay

The assessment of metabolic functions by the cellular ATP content is an established method of measuring cytotoxicity that is essential for screening drugs and determining toxicological safety. As ATP plays a central role in cellular metabolism, the intracellular level of ATP is strictly regulated in normal cells. Furthermore, cell injury results in not only reduced ATP synthesis but also immediate diminution of endogenous ATP levels which is caused by the escape of ATP-converting enzymes (e.g., ATPase) [65]. Therefore, quantification of the intracellular ATP content is crucial for the assessment of the degree of cellular toxicity [66].

5.3 Autophagy assay

Autophagy is a process which is characterized by the formation of double-membraned vesicles called autophagosomes, which isolate the cellular components targeted for devastation and fuse with lysosomes to deliver their content for degradation. Autophagy can be determined by two different methods as direct and indirect. Direct tests are based on the turnover of long-lived proteins and lactate dehydrogenase (LDH) sequestration, while indirect tests include western blot-based assays, fluorescence microscopy-based methods, electron microscopy, and flow cytometry and imaging flow cytometry [67].

5.4 BrdU assay

BrdU is a thymidine analogue used in cell proliferation studies. BrdU in the cell culture medium is incorporated into DNA during DNA synthesis. Once the membrane permeabilization is performed, the cellular incorporation of BrdU can be detected by anti-BrdU-specific antibodies. For this purpose, flow cytometry or immunohistochemistry techniques can be used [68].

5.5 Cell tracking

This is a procedure used to monitor cell movement and location by the implementation of "tracking" probes that pass through the membrane into the cytoplasm and then become membrane impermeable. The "tracking" dyes to be used in this type of experiments should be passed to the daughter cells during multiple generations, but not transferred to the neighboring cells they are in contact [69].

5.6 Gram staining

Although traditionally named "Gram staining," commercial kits for testing cell viability and proliferation now include dyes such as CF®488A WGA, DAPI, Ethidium Homodimer III (EthD-III), etc. in addition to the conventional Gram stain; CF-488A (WGA) stains N-acetylglucosamine structure in the peptidoglycan layer of Gram-positive bacteria with green fluorescence. EthD-III, which is a nucleic acid binding dye, is membrane impermeable and selectively stains the compromised plasma membranes of bacteria with red fluorescence. DAPI, which can pass through the membrane and bind to DNA, stains all bacterial cells in blue [21].

5.7 LDH assay

The cytoplasmic enzyme lactate dehydrogenase is a stable ubiquitous enzyme found in all cells. A key feature of apoptosis, necrosis, and other forms of cellular damage is that the LDH is released into the cell culture, while the plasma membrane is damaged. By using the NADH which is produced in a coupled reaction to reduce a second compound during the conversion of lactate to pyruvate, LDH activity can be quantified. In this protocol, the reduction by NADH of a yellow tetrazolium salt (INT) into a red water-soluble formazan-class dye is quantified at 492 nm absorbance. The amount of formazan occurring in culture is directly proportional to the amount of LDH and, indirectly, to the number of dead or damaged cells in the culture media [70].

5.8 Live/dead staining

Live/dead assay is used for quantification of cell viability using flow cytometry or fluorescence microscopy. This assay utilizes fluorescent dyes to label live and dead cells with a one-step protocol. "Live cell" dye stain intact and viable cells into green. It can pass through the membrane and does not fluoresce until the ester groups in the dye molecule are removed by the intracellular esterases. The excitation (max) and emission (max) are 494 nm and 515 nm, respectively. On the other hand, "dead cell" dye labels cells with damaged plasma membrane into red. It does not have the ability to pass through the plasma membrane and binds to DNA with a high affinity. The degree of the fluorescence emitted by this dye increases up to >30-fold when it is bound to DNA. The excitation (max) and emission (max) are 528 nm and 617 nm, respectively [71, 72].

5.9 Lysosomal staining

These dyes are fluorescent dyes such as "CytoPainter green" or "acridine orange" (AO), which are used to measure lysosomal integrity in proliferating and nonproliferating cells. These lysotropic dyes preferentially accumulate in lysosomes via the lysosome pH gradient. Their fluorescence is significantly increased after they become trapped in lysosomes. These dyes are also useful in cell adhesion, drug resistance, chemotaxis, apoptosis, cell viability, and adherent cell studies [73].

5.10 Membrane potential assay

Membrane potential or membrane voltage refers to the difference of electric charges across a cell membrane. Electrical potential difference across the cell membrane is a novel method to monitor cell death (apoptosis) in single cells. It has been shown that the depolarization of plasma membrane in response to microinjection of cytochrome c into the cytosol is a reliable indicator of apoptotic cell death [74]. The dye used for this assay is a lipophilic and anionic dye that can move across the cytoplasmic membrane of healthy cells, dependent on the membrane potential across the plasma membrane. The fluorescence intensity of the dye increases when the dye is bound to proteins in the cytosol. Following depolarization of the cells, more dye enters the cells, and the increased cellular concentration of dye binding to lipids and proteins results in an increase in fluorescence signal. On the other hand, following hyperpolarization, dye exits the cells, and the decreased intracellular concentration of dye results in a decrease of fluorescence signal. The excitation wavelength of the dye is 488 nm of the argon ion laser [75].

5.11 Mitochondrial staining

Although mitochondrial staining is performed in different compartments of mitochondria, it is usually a test performed on the mitochondrial membrane or mitochondrial matrix. Mitochondrial membrane dyes are cell permeant and accumulate in active mitochondria that have intact membrane potentials. The signal will be bright if the cells under examination are healthy and have functional mitochondria; however, if the mitochondrial membrane potential is lost, the signal will be dimmer or will disappear [76]. In addition to staining the mitochondrial membrane, some dyes stain specific molecules in the mitochondrial matrix. One of them is the "fluorescent mitochondrial hydrogen peroxide indicator" stain, which serves to visualize hydrogen peroxide in the mitochondrial matrix of living cells. This dye gives strong emissions at 528 nm in the presence of H_2O_2. In an in vitro model of Parkinson's disease, it is used to detect the local increases in H_2O_2 [77].

5.12 MTT, XTT, MTS, and WSTs assays

5.12.1 MTT assay

In living cells, MTT (a yellow tetrazole) is reduced to formazan (purple). To convert (dissolve) the insoluble formazan into a colored solution, a solubilization solution (DMSO, acidic ethanol solution, or a solution of sodium dodecyl sulfate in diluted hydrochloric acid) is added. This colored solution can be quantified by measuring its absorbance using a spectrophotometer usually between 500 and 600 nm wavelength. The absorption degree of light depends on the solvent [78].

5.12.2 XTT assay

Due to its higher sensitivity and higher dynamic range, XTT has replaced MTT. Since the formed formazan dye is water-soluble, it eliminates the final solubilization step [79].

5.12.3 MTS assay

MTS, in the presence of phenazine methosulfate (PMS), forms a formazan product which has a max. Absorbance of 490 nm in PBS. The MTS assay is often regarded as a "one-step" MTT assay, since it offers the advantage of adding the reagent directly to the cell culture without any intermediary steps necessary in the MTT assay. Since the intermediary steps remove remnants of colored intermediates in the MTT assay, this advantage, however, makes the MTS assay sensitive to colorimetric interference as these intermediates remain in the one-step MTS assay [80].

5.12.4 WSTs

WSTs (water-soluble tetrazolium salts), a series of other dyes for MTT assays, are designed to give different absorption spectra for the formed formazans. WST-1, particularly WST-8, have advantages over MTT in that they are reduced outside the cells and form a water-soluble formazan. Finally, unlike MTT, WST assays (1) can be read directly, (2) provide stronger signal than MTT, and (3) are less toxic to cells (unlike membrane-permeable MTT, and the resulting insoluble formazan piles up inside the cells) [81].

5.13 In silico prediction of chemical toxicity

A relatively newer discipline, and highly hot topic, which has become increasingly important in recent years, is the computer-aided in silico toxicity prediction of drugs, food additives, or various industrial chemicals for which a previous wet-lab toxicity outcome is available. For this purpose, QSAR, the CAESAR project, and other virtual screening methods such as docking (i.e., AutoDock, Surflex) software have found wide use in the last decade [82–84]. While these software use special parameters (e.g., genetic algorithms), the details of these parameters do not fall into the scope of the main subject of this review article.

6. Conclusion

A thorough understanding of the molecular mechanisms of cell division makes it easy to understand cell death. Cells perform division at the right time according to the chemical signals from their internal and external environment. Aberrations in cell division often induce uncontrolled cell division and result in tumor formation. Here, the importance of cytotoxicity parameters and assays in experimentally normal or abnormally divided cells emerges. Many diseases show a direct correlation with the parameters used to measure the division behavior of cells. Thus, a detailed understanding of the molecular mechanisms of cell division and cell death by cell proliferation and cytotoxicity tests is critical in distinguishing between normal and healthy cells. Another important aspect is the selection of the right cytotoxicity assay when working on different cell death mechanisms such as apoptosis, necrosis, necroptosis, or autophagy. Although they appear to reveal very different death pathways, in fact, cytotoxicity assays mainly target a certain number of cellular compartments (lysosome, membrane, nucleus, cytoplasm, mitochondria). In recent years, with the development of in silico toxicity assessment software, cytotoxicity experiments have been transferred from the laboratory to the computer environment. However, the fact that the details of the intracellular milieu are not completely understood yet still keeps the accuracy of the in silico toxicity estimates at a certain level, and therefore it is logical to anticipate that the wet-lab applications (especially in vitro cytotoxicity tests) to measure cell proliferation and cytotoxicity will continue to be the first choice.

Conflict of interest

The authors declare that they have no competing interests.

Author details

Erman Salih Istifli*, Mehmet Tahir Hüsunet and Hasan Basri Ila
Faculty of Science and Letter, Department of Biology, Çukurova University, Adana, Turkey

*Address all correspondence to: esistifli@cu.edu.tr; ermansalih@gmail.com

IntechOpen

© 2019 The Author(s). Licensee IntechOpen. This chapter is distributed under the terms of the Creative Commons Attribution License (http://creativecommons.org/licenses/by/3.0), which permits unrestricted use, distribution, and reproduction in any medium, provided the original work is properly cited.

References

[1] Marshall WF, Young KD, Swaffer M, Wood E, Nurse P, Kimura A, et al. What determines cell size? BMC Biology. 2012;**10**:101

[2] Kozma SC, Thomas G. Regulation of cell size in growth, development and human disease: PI3K, PKB and S6K. BioEssays. 2002;**24**(1):65-71

[3] Minc N, Burgess D, Chang F. Influence of cell geometry on division-plane positioning. Cell. 2011;**144**(3):414-426

[4] Wagner JK, Setayeshgar S, Sharon LA, Reilly JP, Brun YV. A nutrient uptake role for bacterial cell envelope extensions. Proceedings of the National Academy of Sciences of the United States of America. 2006;**103**(31):11772-11777

[5] Rudland PS, Hallowes RC, Durbin H, Lewis D. Mitogenic activity of pituitary hormones on cell cultures of normal and carcinogen-induced tumor epithelium from rat mammary glands. The Journal of Cell Biology. 1977;**73**(3):561-577

[6] Cook JJ, Haynes KM, Werther GA. Mitogenic effects of growth hormone in cultured human fibroblasts. Evidence for action via local insulin-like growth factor I production. The Journal of Clinical Investigation. 1988;**81**(1):206-212

[7] Tang HY, Lin HY, Zhang S, Davis FB, Davis PJ. Thyroid hormone causes mitogen-activated protein kinase-dependent phosphorylation of the nuclear estrogen receptor. Endocrinology. 2004;**145**(7):3265-3272

[8] Lim S, Kaldis P. Cdks, cyclins and CKIs: Roles beyond cell cycle regulation. Development. 2013;**140**(15):3079-3093

[9] Smith KA. Determining to divide: How do cells decide? Journal of Biological Physics. 2005;**31**(3-4):261-272

[10] Brandt F. 10 Minutes/10 Years: Your Definitive Guide to a Beautiful and Youthful Appearance. 1st Free Press Hardcover ed. Free Press; 2007. https://play.google.com/store/books/details/Frederic_Brandt_10_Minutes_10_Years?id=vrhN-1GVVMAC

[11] Post SG, Binstock RH. The fountain of youth: Cultural, scientific, and ethical perspectives on a biomedical goal. JAMA. 2004;**21**(3):463

[12] Cadart C, Zlotek-Zlotkiewicz E, Le Berre M, Piel M, Matthews HK. Exploring the function of cell shape and size during mitosis. Developmental Cell. 2014;**29**(2):159-169

[13] Ohkura H. Meiosis: An overview of key differences from mitosis. Cold Spring Harbor Perspectives in Biology. 2015;**7**(5):a015859

[14] Ris H, Mirsky AE. The state of the chromosomes in the interphase nucleus. The Journal of General Physiology. 1949;**32**(4):489-502

[15] Dinarina A, Ruiz EJ, O'Loghlen A, Mouron S, Perez L, Nebreda AR. Negative regulation of cell-cycle progression by RINGO/Speedy E. The Biochemical Journal. 2008;**410**(3):535-542

[16] Brugarolas J, Moberg K, Boyd SD, Taya Y, Jacks T, Lees JA. Inhibition of cyclin-dependent kinase 2 by p21 is necessary for retinoblastoma protein-mediated G(1) arrest after gamma-irradiation. Proceedings of the National Academy of Sciences of the United States of America. 1999;**96**(3):1002-1007

[17] Cai ZJ, Liu Q. Cell cycle regulation in treatment of breast cancer. Advances in Experimental Medicine and Biology. 2017;**1026**:251-270

[18] Iness AN, Felthousen J, Ananthapadmanabhan V, Sesay F, Saini S, Guiley KZ, et al. The cell cycle regulatory DREAM complex is disrupted by high expression of oncogenic B-Myb. Oncogene. 2019;**38**(7):1080-1092

[19] Martin LG, Demers GW, Galloway DA. Disruption of the G1/S transition in human papillomavirus type 16 E7-expressing human cells is associated with altered regulation of cyclin E. Journal of Virology. 1998;**72**(2):975-985

[20] Du W, Searle JS. The rb pathway and cancer therapeutics. Current Drug Targets. 2009;**10**(7):581-589

[21] Bacterial Viability and Gram Stain Kit. 2019. Available from: https://biotium.com/product/bacterial-viability-and-gram-stain-kit/ [Accessed: May 26, 2019]

[22] Williams AB, Schumacher B. p53 in the DNA-damage-repair process. Cold Spring Harbor Perspectives in Medicine. 2016;**6**(5):a026070

[23] Hotchkiss RS, Strasser A, McDunn JE, Swanson PE. Mechanisms of disease cell death. The New England Journal of Medicine. 2009;**361**(16):1570-1583

[24] Strasser A, O'Connor L, Dixit VM. Apoptosis signaling. Annual Review of Biochemistry. 2000;**69**:217-245

[25] Delbridge ARD, Valente LJ, Strasser A. The role of the apoptotic machinery in tumor suppression. Cold Spring Harbor Perspectives in Biology. 2012;**4**(11):a008789

[26] Liddell HG, Scott R, Jones HS. A Greek–English Lexicon. Oxford University Press; 1843. https://global.oup.com/academic/product/a-greek-english-lexicon-9780198642268?cc=us&lang=en&

[27] Klionsky DJ. Autophagy revisited: A conversation with Christian de Duve. Autophagy. 2008;**4**(6):740-743

[28] The Nobel Prize in Physiology or Medicine 2016. 2016. Available from: https://www.nobelprize.org/prizes/medicine/2016/summary/ [Accessed: May 15, 2019]

[29] Levine B, Mizushima N, Virgin HW. Autophagy in immunity and inflammation. Nature. 2011;**469**(7330):323-335

[30] Mizushima N, Ohsumi Y, Yoshimori T. Autophagosome formation in mammalian cells. Cell Structure and Function. 2002;**27**(6):421-429

[31] Cesen MH, Pegan K, Spes A, Turk B. Lysosomal pathways to cell death and their therapeutic applications. Experimental Cell Research. 2012;**318**(11):1245-1251

[32] Shang LB, Chen S, Du FH, Li S, Zhao LP, Wang XD. Nutrient starvation elicits an acute autophagic response mediated by Ulk1 dephosphorylation and its subsequent dissociation from AMPK. Proceedings of the National Academy of Sciences of the United States of America. 2011;**108**(12):4788-4793

[33] Maiuri MC, Zalckvar E, Kimchi A, Kroemer G. Self-eating and self-killing: Crosstalk between autophagy and apoptosis. Nature Reviews. Molecular Cell Biology. 2007;**8**(9):741-752

[34] Tavassoly I, Parmar J, Shajahan-Haq AN, Clarke R, Baumann WT, Tyson JJ. Dynamic modeling of the interaction between autophagy and apoptosis in mammalian cells. CPT: Pharmacometrics & Systems Pharmacology. 2015;**4**(4):263-272

[35] Degenhardt K, Mathew R, Beaudoin B, Bray K, Anderson D, Chen G, et al. Autophagy promotes tumor

[36] Proskuryakov SY, Konoplyannikov AG, Gabai VL. Necrosis: A specific form of programmed cell death? Experimental Cell Research. 2003;**283**(1):1-16

[37] Kasper DL, Zaleznik DF. Gas Gangrene, Antibiotic Associated Colitis, and Other Clostridial Infections. New York: McGraw-Hill, Medical Pub. Division; 2001. pp. 922-927. www.scienceopen.com

cell survival and restricts necrosis, inflammation, and tumorigenesis. Cancer Cell. 2006;**10**(1):51-64

[38] Rock KL, Kono H. The inflammatory response to cell death. Annual Review of Pathology. 2008;**3**:99-126

[39] Adigun R, Basit H, Murray J. Necrosis, Cell (Liquefactive, Coagulative, Caseous, Fat, Fibrinoid, and Gangrenous). Treasure Island, FL: StatPearls; 2019

[40] Dhuriya YK, Sharma D. Necroptosis: A regulated inflammatory mode of cell death. Journal of Neuroinflammation. 2018;**15**(1):199

[41] Riss TL, Moravec RA. Use of multiple assay endpoints to investigate the effects of incubation time, dose of toxin, and plating density in cell-based cytotoxicity assays. Assay and Drug Development Technologies. 2004;**2**(1):51-62

[42] Hyesun HO, Surapaneni S, Hui JY. Preclinical development of oncology drugs. In: Faqi AS, editor. A Comprehensive Guide to Toxicology in Preclinical Drug Development. London: Academic Press; 2013. pp. 543-565

[43] Linder R, Bernheimer AW. Action of bacterial cytotoxins on normal mammalian cells and cells with altered membrane lipid composition. Toxicon. 1984;**22**(4):641-651

[44] Nappi AJ, Ottaviani E. Cytotoxicity and cytotoxic molecules in invertebrates. BioEssays. 2000;**22**(5):469-480

[45] Aktories K, Barbieri JT. Bacterial cytotoxins: Targeting eukaryotic switches. Nature Reviews. Microbiology. 2005;**3**(5):397-410

[46] Davidson JF, Schiestl RH. Cytotoxic and genotoxic consequences of heat stress are dependent on the presence of oxygen in *Saccharomyces cerevisiae*. Journal of Bacteriology. 2001;**183**(15):4580-4587

[47] Saad AH, Hahn GM. Ultrasound enhanced drug toxicity on Chinese hamster ovary cells in vitro. Cancer Research. 1989;**49**(21):5931-5934

[48] Mariglia J, Momin S, Coe IR, Karshafian R. Analysis of the cytotoxic effects of combined ultrasound, microbubble and nucleoside analog combinations on pancreatic cells in vitro. Ultrasonics. 2018;**89**:110-117

[49] Bahadar H, Maqbool F, Niaz K, Abdollahi M. Toxicity of nanoparticles and an overview of current experimental models. Iranian Biomedical Journal. 2016;**20**(1):1-11

[50] Walker PMB. The mitotic index and interphase processes. The Journal of Experimental Biology. 1954;**31**:8-15

[51] Van't Hof J, Kovacs CJ. Mitotic delay in two biochemically different G1 cell populations in cultured roots of pea (*Pisum sativum*). Radiation Research. 1970;**44**(3):700-712

[52] Graña E. Mitotic index. In: Sánchez-Moreiras AM, Reigosa MJ, editors. Advances in Plant Ecophysiology Techniques. Switzerland: Springer; 2018. pp. 231-240

[53] Sharma S, Vig AP. Antigenotoxic effects of Indian mustard *Brassica juncea* (L.) Czern aqueous seeds extract against

mercury (Hg) induced genotoxicity. Scientific Research and Essays. 2012;7(13):1385-1392

[54] Evseeva TI, Geras'kin SA, Shuktomova II. Genotoxicity and toxicity assay of water sampled from a radium production industry storage cell territory by means of Allium-test. Journal of Environmental Radioactivity. 2003;68(3):235-248

[55] Al-Ahmadi S. Effects of organic insecticides, Kingbo and Azdar 10 EC, on mitotic chromosomes in root tip cells of *Allium cepa*. International Journal of Genetics and Molecular Biology. 2013;5(5):64-70

[56] Borah SP, Talukdar J. Studies on the phytotoxic effects of extract of castor seed (*Ricinus communis* L.). Cytologia. 2002;67:235-243

[57] Madaan N, Mudgal V. Phytotoxic effects of selenium on the accessions of wheat and safflower. Research Journal of Environmental Sciences. 2011;5(1):82-87

[58] Ha SY, Choi M, Lee T, Park CK. The prognostic role of mitotic index in hepatocellular carcinoma patients after curative hepatectomy. Cancer Research and Treatment. 2016;48(1):180-189

[59] Gaffney EV 2nd, Venz-Williamson TL, Hutchinson G, Biggs PJ, Nelson KM. Relationship of standardized mitotic indices to other prognostic factors in breast cancer. Archives of Pathology & Laboratory Medicine. 1996;120(5):473-477

[60] Meyer JS, Cosatto E, Graf HP. Mitotic index of invasive breast carcinoma. Achieving clinically meaningful precision and evaluating tertial cutoffs. Archives of Pathology & Laboratory Medicine. 2009;133(11):1826-1833

[61] Fenech M, Kirsch-Volders M. RE: Insensitivity of the in vitro cytokinesis-block micronucleus assay with human lymphocytes for the detection of DNA damage present at the start of the cell culture (Mutagenesis, 27, 743-747, 2012). Mutagenesis. 2013;28(3):367-369

[62] Ionescu ME, Ciocirlan M, Becheanu G, Nicolaie T, Ditescu C, Teiusanu AG, et al. Nuclear division index may predict neoplastic colorectal lesions. Maedica (Buchar). 2011;6(3):173-178

[63] Fenech M. The in vitro micronucleus technique. Mutation Research. 2000;455(1-2):81-95

[64] Oancea M, Mazumder S, Crosby ME, Almasan A. Apoptosis assays. Methods in Molecular Medicine. 2006;129:279-290

[65] Imamura H, Nhat KP, Togawa H, Saito K, Iino R, Kato-Yamada Y, et al. Visualization of ATP levels inside single living cells with fluorescence resonance energy transfer-based genetically encoded indicators. Proceedings of the National Academy of Sciences of the United States of America. 2009;106(37):15651-15656

[66] Lee MS, Park WS, Kim YH, Ahn WG, Kwon SH, Her S. Intracellular ATP assay of live cells using PTD-conjugated luciferase. Sensors (Basel). 2012;12(11):15628-15637

[67] Orhon I, Reggiori F. Assays to monitor autophagy progression in cell cultures. Cell. 2017;6(3):E20

[68] B.D. Pharmingen. Bromodeoxyuridine (BrdU). 2014. Available from: http://www.bdbiosciences.com/ds/pm/tds/550891.pdf [Accessed: May 26, 2019]

[69] Cell Tracking. 2019. Available from: https://www.thermofisher.com/tr/en/home/life-science/cell-analysis/cell-tracing-tracking-and-morphology/cell-tracking.html [Accessed: May 26, 2019]

[70] Kumar P, Nagarajan A, Uchil PD. Analysis of cell viability by the lactate dehydrogenase assay. Cold Spring Harbor Protocols. 2018;**2018**(6):pdb prot095497

[71] Amirikia M, Ali Jorsaraei SG, Ali Shariatzadeh SM, Mehranjani MS. Differentiation of stem cells from the apical papilla into osteoblasts by the elastic modulus of porous silk fibroin scaffolds. Biologicals. 2019;**57**:1-8

[72] Bahari L, Bein A, Yashunsky V, Braslavsky I. Directional freezing for the cryopreservation of adherent mammalian cells on a substrate. PLoS One. 2018;**13**(2):e0192265

[73] Lysosomal Staining Reagent—Green—Cytopainter (ab176826). 2019. Available from: https://www.abcam.com/lysosomal-staining-reagent-green-cytopainter-ab176826.html [Accessed: May 26, 2019]

[74] Bhuyan AK, Varshney A, Mathew MK. Resting membrane potential as a marker of apoptosis: Studies on Xenopus oocytes microinjected with cytochrome c. Cell Death and Differentiation. 2001;**8**(1):63-69

[75] Measuring Membrane Potential using the FLIPR® Membrane Potential Assay Kit on Fluorometric Imaging Plate Reader (FLIPR®) Systems. 2019. Available from: https://www.moleculardevices.com/en/assets/app-note/reagents/measuring-membrane-potential-using-flipr-membrane-potential-assay-kit-on-flipr#gref [Accessed: May 26, 2019]

[76] ThermoFisher. Functional Mitochondrial Staining Protocol. 2019. Available from: https://www.thermofisher.com/tr/en/home/life-science/cell-analysis/cell-analysis-learning-center/molecular-probes-school-of-fluorescence/imaging-basics/protocols-troubleshooting/protocols/functional-mitochondrial-staining.html [Accessed: May 26, 2019]

[77] TOCRIS. MitoPY1. 2019. Available from: https://www.tocris.com/about-tocris [Accessed: May 26, 2019]

[78] Mosmann T. Rapid colorimetric assay for cellular growth and survival: Application to proliferation and cytotoxicity assays. Journal of Immunological Methods. 1983;**65**(1-2):55-63

[79] Kuhn DM, Balkis M, Chandra J, Mukherjee PK, Ghannoum MA. Uses and limitations of the XTT assay in studies of *Candida* growth and metabolism. Journal of Clinical Microbiology. 2003;**41**(1):506-508

[80] Cory AH, Owen TC, Barltrop JA, Cory JG. Use of an aqueous soluble tetrazolium/formazan assay for cell growth assays in culture. Cancer Communications. 1991;**3**(7):207-212

[81] Yin LM, Wei Y, Wang Y, Xu YD, Yang YQ. Long term and standard incubations of WST-1 reagent reflect the same inhibitory trend of cell viability in rat airway smooth muscle cells. International Journal of Medical Sciences. 2013;**10**(1):68-72

[82] Yang H, Sun L, Li W, Liu G, Tang Y. In silico prediction of chemical toxicity for drug design using machine learning methods and structural alerts. Frontiers in Chemistry. 2018;**6**:30

[83] Cassano A, Manganaro A, Martin T, Young D, Piclin N, Pintore M, et al. CAESAR models for developmental toxicity. Chemistry Central Journal. 2010;**4**(Suppl 1):S4

[84] Makarova K, Siudem P, Zawada K, Kurkowiak J. Screening of toxic effects of bisphenol a and products of its degradation: Zebrafish (*Danio rerio*) embryo test and molecular docking. Zebrafish. 2016;**13**(5):466-474

Lightning Source UK Ltd.
Milton Keynes UK
UKHW052142101221
395337UK00001B/20